THE LINKED DIET

*Connecting Mindset, Digestive Health and
Weight Loss for Your Best Self*

LAURA KOPEC

BALBOA.
PRESS

A DIVISION OF HAY HOUSE

Balboa Press books may be ordered through booksellers or by contacting:

Balboa Press
A Division of Hay House
1663 Liberty Drive
Bloomington, IN 47403
www.balboapress.com
1 (877) 407-4847

Because of the dynamic nature of the Internet, any web addresses or links contained in this book may have changed since publication and may no longer be valid. The views expressed in this work are solely those of the author and do not necessarily reflect the views of the publisher, and the publisher hereby disclaims any responsibility for them.

The author of this book does not dispense medical advice or prescribe the use of any technique as a form of treatment for physical, emotional, or medical problems without the advice of a physician, either directly or indirectly. The intent of the author is only to offer information of a general nature to help you in your quest for emotional and spiritual well-being. In the event you use any of the information in this book for yourself, which is your constitutional right, the author and the publisher assume no responsibility for your actions.

Any people depicted in stock imagery provided by Thinkstock are models, and such images are being used for illustrative purposes only. Certain stock imagery © Thinkstock.

Print information available on the last page.

ISBN: 978-1-5043-5980-1 (sc)
ISBN: 978-1-5043-5979-5 (e)

Balboa Press rev. date: 07/05/2016

This book is dedicated to my father who is no longer present on this earth. His health journey was profound. He is forever an inspiration to me to help others with their weight and their health.

TABLE OF CONTENTS

ACKNOWLEDGEMENTS

I would like to thank each and every woman who has come into my office struggling to the find the solution to their weight loss and teaching me to dig deeper for the answers.

I would like to thank the many health care professionals that have recommended me to provide educational support to their patients. Thank you for your trust and recognition.

I am blessed for my precious family that is so very valuable to me, especially the support of Jerry Kopec, Dan Kopec, Marc Cook, Pat Loewy, John and Diane Kopec, and Kevin Kopec.

A special thank you to my children Sierra Thain, Luke Thain and Eden Orchard.

I am thankful to my girlfriends: Beverly Wells, Tamara Crawford, Kari Berry, and Alex Hyman who believe in me and inspire me to keep going no matter what life brings.

I would like to thank Anita Battista for her expertise, her guidance and support.

Thank you to Karimen Montero and Sandy Gluckman for their contributions to this project.

Thank you to Hillary Jarrard, Samantha Naidoo, Melissa Irvin and Dannah Blumenau for becoming more than clients through the years.

A special thank you to Amanda Orchard Fernandez in admiration for her determination.

I am grateful to see the change in the general population. More and more educated individuals want something different; as a result, there is growing support of functional practitioners and educators who believe there is a different path toward total health and wellness.

A NOTE TO THE READER

The information in this book is provided to educate the reader. Educational information in this book is for adults only and is not intended for use with children. Any decision involving the treatment of an illness or condition should be made only after consulting a physician or health care practitioner of the reader's choice. Neither this nor any book can guarantee complete absence of disease nor substitute professional medical care or treatment. The information contained in this book is not intended to serve as a replacement for professional medical advice. Any use of the information in this book is at the reader's discretion. The author and the publisher specifically disclaim any and all liability arising directly or indirectly from the use or application of any information contained in this book. A health care professional should be consulted regarding the reader's specific situation. The client names have been eliminated in specific stories to protect their privacy.

INTRODUCTION

After years of fad diets, appetite suppressants and prefab meals, weight loss is still one of the most significant challenges for many adults and now many children. Many of us are buying into numerous misconceptions about weight loss. We take pills we so desperately want to work without changing our food choices, or we count calories without getting permanent results. We drink diet drinks and eat fat-free junk food believing these are important, strategic steps to losing weight. These and more misconceptions add up to limited results. Far too many typical diets have been proven to fail at long-term results. Yet, we continue to search for the magic pill, the quick fix, or the instant solution to being overweight. And it continues to be elusive and is only made more elusive by society's standards.

Our media perpetuates a body image that has very little to do with healthy eating, overall wellness or true self-esteem. We are bombarded with retouched photo images leading us to believe we are flawed. Adults obsess with youthful glow and body image. The aging process is not respected or admired. Unless you can "reverse the signs of aging," you are asked to be ashamed. The focus is on finding ways to halt the aging process instead of aging gracefully and healthy; as a result, we continually fall short of promoting a healthy body image.

After years of working with clients through their weight loss successes and failures, it is apparent to me that the powerful combination of a healthy weight loss mindset added to individualized nutrition is necessary for long-term, healthy weight loss success. Clients with a healthy mindset were able to stay committed to their plan and achieve tremendous, life-changing results in addition to reaching their weight goals. The clients with an unhealthy mindset often lost interest with the plan and ultimately did not see the results they hoped for. There is a lot more to actual weight loss than explaining to someone what they should or should not eat. A healthy weight is about more than a diet; it is an intricate blend of health-promoting nutrition and a healthy mindset. Suddenly, a healthy and successful weight loss plan that included what other plans were missing came into view. This plan would connect true health and wellness with weight loss by:

- Dispelling misconceptions and empowering a new way to think about and approach weight loss and diets.

- Being clear about basics such as calories.
- Attending to the uniqueness of the individual, especially how his/her body responds to food.
- Considering the effects of your personal digestive system imbalances, detoxification systems, and stress have on weight loss.
- Provide optimal food lists, menu plans and recipes that strengthen your digestive health based on your personal symptoms.

If you hope for long-term weight loss and health, you cannot overlook any one aspect of your eating, including how you think about food and your dieting goals. Digestion begins in the brain due to the judgments we make about food before it even goes into our mouths. I believe it is more than your personal view on food choices; it is also your thinking about why you eat. If you address your current thinking and make changes in the way you view yourself, food and the world around you, results can be more consistent and permanent.

A chain is only as strong as its weakest link. I suggest that your weight loss chain is weak because it is missing fundamental links that provide real and lasting strength to the whole chain. If you have tried a variety of diets without success, have achieved initial success only to stop midway to your goal, or put the weight you lost right back on, then I wrote this book for you. Think about your previous weight loss attempts. Write one or two of your previous goals here:

_____

_____

Did your goals focus mainly on results of what your body would look like? It's very important to have healthy conversations with yourself about weight by using words that focus on personal health. Talking about a healthy weight should be very different from talking about body image. A great first step is eliminating image-conscious words like *fat*, *skinny*, *size*, *inches*, and *pounds* from descriptions of yourself, your goals and your progress toward those goals. Talking about your own health and wellness and *feeling* your best is motivating self-talk. Use the questions below to help shift your mind's focus to goals other than a number on a scale or a desired waist size. Your goals will then more likely reflect the level of health you desire, instead of a skewed or media-driven body image.

"Am I the best version of myself I can be?" _____

"Am I happy with my weight relative to my height?" _____

"What 5 things would my best self be able to do that my current weight prevents or hinders?" (List more than 5 if more come to mind.)

_____

_____

_____

_____

_____

"Is my current weight contributing to any of my health issues?" _____
"What would life be like if some of my health issues improved?"

_____

_____

_____

Now, look at your answers. Can you see a new kind of goal that focuses on your ability to live life to its fullest instead of living life as a slave to the scale or to a "perfect," media-driven body image?

This new perspective is only the beginning of creating a hopeful, healthy mindset. While reading this book and completing the suggested activities, you will be equipped to more fully understand and add the missing links to your weight loss chain. These missing links work together to improve your digestive health and adjust your current mindset. This powerful combination will help your body respond differently to food and help you craft a way of thinking that helps you stay committed to your health and well-being. This is the ultimate weight loss program; this is _The Linked Diet: Connecting Mindset, Digestive Health and Weight Loss for Your Best Self._

CHAPTER 1

THE MISSING LINKS TO WEIGHT LOSS

As you hopefully began to see in the introduction of this book, real weight loss is not just about the number of pounds lost. It is also about making significant changes to your body and your health that make keeping the pounds off a reality. A good plan that includes weight loss goals with positive strategies for eating and thinking will help you truly move from a short-term diet success to a committed lifestyle plan that allows your best physical self to shine through. In fact, individuals who achieve weight loss, most likely did so because they strived for a lifestyle change instead of just following a diet. Their weight loss plan was made up of all the links necessary and each link was strong.

In order to embrace a good life program for permanent change to your weight and your health, you need a good understanding of *why* a new kind of thinking and a new kind of plan is necessary. Old thinking and diet plans, which focus on your body's image more than your body's health, will inevitably keep you looking to new versions of the same weight loss failure. Your weight loss chain will remain lacking and weak for two reasons: (1) Every variation of the old chain contains links that are weakened by a lack of true understanding of each link's impact, and (2) Every variation is missing links that, if present, would connect the impact your diet has on vital aspects of health and weight loss success. These weak and missing links include:

- The consumption of too little calories while you are dieting,
- Failure to look at the quality of your food choices versus viewing calories of all foods as equal in value,
- Failure to look at your digestive health relative to the food you choose to eat,
- Failure to look at your stress and the emotional side of your eating,
- Failure to connect your weight loss goals to your life goals or priorities,
- Not establishing accountability and or a support system during your journey.

1

A new plan with a new way of thinking can be the first significant step to making permanent health and weight changes. Let's consider each link's impact on your success.

Consuming Too Little Calories

Let's consider a typical weak link of weight loss – misunderstanding the effect of calories in weight loss and thus consuming too little calories. Yes, you can actually hinder weight loss, not to mention good health, by eating too few calories. If you are like most Americans, this radical idea goes against everything you know about weight loss. Most of my clients are absolutely shocked when I tell them to *stop counting calories.* This goes against what we have been taught all our lives about losing weight. But significant caloric restriction may actually cause you to gain weight or may be the reason you put the weight back on after reaching your goal.

When you eat too few calories you may be causing your body to freak out a little bit. Your body starts to "think" that food may be scarce and it is in danger of starving because it is not getting enough calories to support the body's basic nutritional needs and health. The body then takes preventative measures by slowing down to reserve the few calories it is getting. As a result, the body may alter its own metabolic rate which hinders its ability to burn calories. This slowed metabolic rate is the body's attempt at survival because when you do not meet your nutritional needs, the body kicks into a "starvation mode." When this happens during the "diet phase," you may or may not lose weight. The big problem is once you stop the diet and return to normal eating. When you alter your caloric burn rate and return to "normal" eating you are now eating too many calories to support the slowed caloric burn rate. So now, even though you have returned to regular calorie consumption, it is too much for the body to burn. You put on the weight you just lost.

Does this mean you have to stay in your previous diet phase for the rest of your life? No. What it means is that severe caloric restriction to lose weight is dangerous and costly to the body; and if you have already completed a diet phase of severe caloric restriction, then a very slow increase of calories is called for to prevent an instant return to your previous eating style and a quick regain of the pounds lost.

Consuming the Wrong Kind of Calories

The next diet misconception believes counting calories alone will bring the desired results. This method pays no attention to the *kind* of calorie that is most beneficial. When the caloric focus is on quantity and not quality, long term results are nonexistent. The reality is *if you eat a little bit of a bad thing, it is still a bad thing. On the other hand, a nutrient dense food should never be restricted.* When the body ultimately craves and needs nutrient-rich foods, limiting calories from nutrient-rich food is still starving the body's true needs and depriving you of the ultimate goal of good health and wellbeing. But many of us gravitate to this kind of diet, so we can still eat foods that satisfy cravings. As you will see, these cravings result from foods that contain ingredients that have, through continued overuse, tricked our brains and changed our body's chemical makeup to "need" them. This is not easy to overcome, but it is possible.

Most of us are driven by certain addictive tastes such as salty, sweet and fatty tasting foods. When we consistently consume large amounts of processed foods containing high amounts of sodium, fat and sugar our taste buds become altered. We then find we are continually seeking out those foods to satisfy the altered taste buds.

Many clients walk into my office with health issues and swear they do not understand how they can be unhealthy. After all, they grocery shop exclusively at a health food store! I then have to give them a reality check. Even in health food stores, you can find the equivalent "bad" food choices. Even though these foods are processed without a single chemical, which is a great improvement, they still contain vast amounts of sodium, sugar and fat. They simply managed a dietary change from inexpensive and truly harmful, chemical-ridden foods to expensive, but still processed, foods. If your diet is missing a certain quota of whole, unadulterated food, then you will fail in reaching your true health and weight goals.

The body craves and runs on nutrients from whole and unprocessed foods. What does this mean for someone trying to lose weight? The bottom line is the more nutrient-dense your food is, the faster the burn rate. Foods containing high amounts of nutrients are used by the body more efficiently and more effectively. Foods that satisfy our altered taste buds' cravings are not used by the body, and thus are very slow to metabolize and very harmful to our success. In some cases, these foods need to be eliminated; in others, strict portion control is necessary.

The overall goal of weight loss should be significant consumption of the foods with greater nutrient density, which translates to you as a higher metabolic rate, and less or none at all of the nutrient-deprived foods that equal empty calories and are slow to burn. Consider this example of an apple versus an apple pastry. A calorie-counting diet states that a whole apple or one 100-calorie apple pastry is an acceptable snack. Which one makes better sense to eat? Though the pastry may seem to satisfy the taste buds' craving for something sweet, it is laden with ingredients the body will not use. The whole apple, on the other hand, will be burned more efficiently because the body will use its nutrients. The apple will also actually help satisfy the craving and control your appetite.

The form of the food also has a tremendous impact on how your body handles the food. A whole orange, is faster to burn than pasteurized orange juice. A complete balance of live enzymes with soluble and insoluble fiber is contained within a whole orange. This allows the body to metabolize the orange much more efficiently than the juice that has no enzyme activity and may, in fact, have more naturally occurring sugar than the whole orange.

Failure to Address Personal Digestive Health

A weight loss link almost always missing, and thus rarely considered, is the body's own communication about the food it is receiving. Many of our symptoms and health issues stem from straying too far off our body's optimal path for too long, and our digestive systems are trying to let us know how to get back on that path. By understanding how your individual digestive system responds to various foods, you can interpret your body's language of symptoms to know how to restore digestive health. It is then that you are benefiting from allowing your body to be an additional accountability partner.

Typical diets recommend caloric restriction with very little consideration to digestive health. Without restoring the way your body handles food, most diets will not get the job done. Some of your symptoms will go away with a healthier weight, but some will not. A good dietary plan will be a good fit for your digestive individuality. Each and every one of us is unique by design, a creation of our genetics, our home environment, our birth order, our diet, our culture, our stress and our sleep habits to name a few. As a result, a one-size-fits-all diet plan can be very unsatisfying to anyone whose individuality does not really fit with that diet.

Failure to Address Stress and the Emotional Side of Eating

The next missing link is failure to address stress and the emotional side of eating while changing what and how you eat. This book contains clear cut strategies and exercises to help in this area, so you will have tools. Here is why it is so vital to have these tools. Many of you overeat to fill a greater need. You may be eating to fill a void that exists inside you. The void is valid. If you are filling an emotional void with food, then depriving yourself of food, as in a typical diet, simultaneously increases your emotional needs and the likelihood that you will give up on your diet plan. You cannot ignore your emotional needs. Unless you learn to fill the void with something other than food, changes in your weight will be short-lived or not happen at all.

Typical diets rarely address this issue much less provide you with alternative tools to fulfill yourself emotionally. Decreasing your calories or changing your diet *without* addressing the emotional eating will only leave you very unsatisfied; possibly further contributing to depression or feelings of sadness or an emptiness that cannot be filled. This book will not only change your view of food and teach you how to eat; it also aims to help you learn how to think differently about eating itself so you can avoid eating out of pure emotion.

Establishing Weight Loss Goals That Work with Your Life Priorities

Each link of the weight loss chain must be in place for complete success. If you fail to look at the previous link regarding stress and emotional eating, then your efforts to establish this link regarding your priorities will likely fail. If these two are not strongly linked together, complete success will be much harder to come by. *You have the power to make these two links build each other up or tear each other down.*

No matter what we say to ourselves, we always have the time, money and energy for the things that are most important to us. And we pay hardly any attention to the things that are not that important to us. There is no right or wrong to what is important to you and what you prioritize. It is your life, and the way you craft your priorities is one of the things that make you truly unique. That having been said, your health has to be important to you in order to improve it, or you will not stay focused on the work involved in being healthy. If your health is not important to you yet, that is okay. You cannot just wake up one day and decide to make it important without some help. This book will teach you how to align your health and wellness with the areas that are most important to you.

Understanding Accountability and a Support System

The last missing link in weight loss is accountability and support. Accountability is the force that helps us stay committed to any plan or goal. Typically a doctor, a weight loss counselor, a nutritionist, a boot camp instructor or even a friend or family member attempts to fill this role. Some of the best results for weight loss happen in a confined setting where accountability and support are enforced. A lot of these facilities are very expensive and time-consuming. These facilities and professionals may not be available to you, or many of you reading this simply will not have the time, money or means for a live-in, supervised environment. And many times friends and family, though well-intentioned and helpful, are just not enough. That should not mean that anyone living at home cannot lose weight. It just means there has to be a solid plan. You may be used to tracking your weight and reporting what foods were eaten in order to count calories. This book will take you on a different path for holding yourself accountable.

Let's review. The missing links are the consumption of too little calories while dieting, focusing on the wrong kind of calorie consideration and continued "bad" food consumption, failure to look at your personal digestive health and what that means for your food choices, failure to look at stress and the emotional side of eating, failure to establish weight loss goals and actions that are in line with your priorities, and not creating enough accountability and support.

As you can see, a new weight loss plan is necessary. That plan is the Linked Diet. It has been created for you to get faster and better results. Every link is present and strategies for increasing each link's strength are included so that you can:

1. Eat enough calories to support your mental and physical activity,
2. Consider quality of calories over quantity of calories and make good food choices abundant over food choices that are nutritionally void,
3. Incorporate food choices that support the most overlooked link in your diet—your digestive health,
4. Examine the emotional side of eating and begin to use provided tools to help you cope,
5. Use the strategies provided for making your health a priority in your life,
6. Use the tools given for staying accountable.

I'm excited you are taking this journey! You are on your way to experiencing your best self. You can do it!

CHAPTER 2

NEW THINKING, NEW PLAN

Many of my weight loss clients bring up exercise apologetically believing that, if they only exercised, they would not be sitting in my office in the first place. Exercise has its place, but it is not the single greatest reason we lose weight. In fact, weight loss is 80% what you eat and 20% what you do.

On the surface exercise makes sense, burn more calories than you consume. While this is true to some degree, the theory of burn more than you consume ignores some fundamental rules about food and its effect on individuals, especially older individuals. A good exercise program can help you shed the pounds faster than without one, but *every exercise program without a good dietary plan, will not give you complete results.* You will run yourself in circles trying to get faster results. You may even find yourself gaining weight once you begin an exercise program if you have not included a proper dietary plan. Implementing a good diet plan first and then adding exercise is a much better strategy.

Once you understand the need for a good dietary plan first, the next question is what to eat. Every person has a unique makeup influenced by genetics, lifestyle factors, and how his or her body responds to food. As a result, what works for one person may not work for another. Ultimately, you want a diet that enhances your physical performance, helps you meet your fitness goals, *and* helps you meet your health goals. Let's face it, if you follow a diet that helps you lose the pounds, but you still suffer constipation, chronic headaches and/or other bothersome symptoms are you truly fit?

Your metabolism is based on not just what you eat, but how your body deals with food. Your personal diet plan should help you restore balance to your digestive system's ability to efficiently digest food and detoxify the body naturally. The questionnaire in the next chapter helps you discover the weaknesses in your digestion and detoxification. This will point you toward your personal food plan. You will then be given a specific list of foods that are best for you to eat as well as a list of foods you should avoid so that your efforts will not be derailed. You will also find some basic supplement suggestions that can enhance these food choices. By following your food plan, you will find food that works for you instead of against you.

Once you follow your food plan, you will feel better, perform better and put yourself in a better position to lose the weight. Even if weight loss is not your primary goal, if your goal is to tone your body, the Linked Diet can help you change some of those pounds to lean muscle weight when combined with a good exercise program. The reason the Linked Diet works is that it takes into consideration all the elements necessary.

There are some common nutritional considerations necessary for every food plan. Let's consider protein first. A diet containing adequate amounts of quality protein is essential for building muscle, muscle synthesis, and muscle recovery. Many people understand the importance of protein but fail to consider the quality of protein. You really have to pay attention to the quality of protein you are eating. Whole-food protein such as eggs, chicken, turkey and fish are better sources of protein than luncheon meats, hot dogs, and other processed meats. Some protein powders can be very difficult for the body to handle because they may be too quickly absorbed and are not as good as whole foods. The Paleo Diet is an example of an excellent protein dominant diet. However, many people I work with misunderstand the Paleo Diet and wind up eating far too much animal protein at one time.

What you combine with protein is just as important as the quality of the protein. Refined carbohydrates combined with protein, such as in a turkey sandwich, will slow the absorption of the protein and thus your metabolism. Instead of refined carbohydrates, combine your protein with a good vegetable carbohydrate, like salmon filet with steamed broccoli to make sure the absorption of the protein is smooth and efficient. When you eat vegetables and leafy greens with protein you are also balancing the underlying acidity of protein. Without watching the amount of acidity in your diet from animal proteins, grains, most vegetable oils and sugar, you are not only slowing your metabolism; but also increasing the inflammation in your body. Inflammation can make exercise very uncomfortable and increase your risk of injury.

And yes, you read that right. Broccoli is a carbohydrate. The term *carbohydrate* encompasses more than just the refined carbohydrates such as breads, pasta, and crackers. Vegetables, along with fruit, are good carbohydrates, and they are absolutely essential to weight loss, injury prevention and protein absorption. These carbohydrates are key to making you lose weight and feel great! The idea of eating the proper amount of carbohydrates is not often a consideration when trying to lose weight. Anyone who says they are "cutting out the carbs" or eating "low carb" has skewed thinking about what a carbohydrate is and how important it is to get high-quality carbohydrates in the form of fruits and vegetables. If you limit your refined carbohydrates and processed food, but fail to increase *good* carbohydrates; then you are not getting real results. You need to make sure the quality of carbohydrates is good enough to support your health and fitness goals.

Fats also have to be a consideration. The quality of fat is important since certain fats are more inflammatory that others. If there is inflammation, your body is not running as efficiently as without inflammation. Thus, your body may not be losing weight as quickly as it could, and it may not be toning or building muscle as quickly as it could. Quite frankly, if you are experiencing inflammation of any kind in any part of your body, then any kind of diet or exercise program isn't going to feel very good. As a result, your motivation may be undermined. Poor quality fat is not the only source of food that may contribute to inflammation. Other food sources such as gluten and sugars can also contribute to inflammation in the body. Significantly reducing or eliminating these foods, based on your dietary type, may enhance your body's performance both in weight loss and in health; thus your motivation to continue to strive toward your health goals will be strengthened.

Until now, the majority of diets employ a system of counting calories or measuring portions. This is such a small piece of the big picture. Knowing the difference between an empty calorie and a nutrient-dense food is essential to understanding the effects of food on your body. The nutrients in an apple or banana are not anywhere close to the same as the nutrients in a low calorie breakfast bar. This cannot be stressed enough as a fundamental rule to faster weight loss—*the quality of carbohydrate is essential.* As mentioned earlier, the metabolic rate of food has to be considered in order to get the fastest results possible.

The next chapter provides you with the tools to help discover your individual food needs. By eating according to your Linked Type, you are taking a huge step in achieving true weight loss goals. The information you learn about yourself and the food you eat will help balance your digestion and detoxification in order for you to keep those unwanted pounds from coming back. Not only can you potentially lose weight, but you may also find relief from many symptoms that have plagued you for years as a result of eating food that did not fit your personal digestive profile.

CHAPTER 3

LINKING YOUR DIGESTION AND YOUR DIETARY TYPE

One of the most significant missing links to successful weight loss and personal health is identifying the phase in your digestive cycle that is the weakest. The body is ultimately one whole system, and the ultimate goal is not only to lose the weight, but to also become a healthier version of you. In my professional experience, each of our body's digestive cycle has one predominantly weak area that allows for digestive imbalances that in turn affect other systems or areas of the body because of the interconnectedness of the entire bodily system. The area where your digestion is most weak will determine which foods will (1) create more inflammation or other issues in your body and (2) slow your progress should you eat these foods, no matter how harmless or healthy these foods may seem or even be for others. So again, while the goal is to eat healthy and improve your overall health and wellness, your specific digestive weak link will dictate which foods will allow you the fastest results.

Our digestive system basically starts in the brain with our perception of foods. This can trigger an actual physical response. For example, the thought of certain foods can make our mouth water or our stomach go queasy. The brain is a powerful phase in the digestive process. The next phase is the mouth. Chewing food releases saliva that has powerful enzymes to help break down carbohydrates. Food then travels to the stomach which is mostly responsible for the breakdown of proteins and of minerals, followed by the small intestine where most of the absorption of our nutrients occurs through tiny hair-like fibers called *villi*. Other phases include the liver and gall bladder which helps us break down fats and the large intestine where we eliminate waste.

By identifying your Linked Diet Type and following the food plan for your Linked Type, you will be guided to a customized eating plan that will help strengthen the digestive weaknesses and resolve nutritional imbalances that may be interfering in your ability to lose weight. When you eat foods that strengthen your digestive system, you are eating foods that strengthen your metabolism. When you strengthen digestion and metabolism you increase your chances of losing weight and feeling better.

Identifying Your Linked Type

1. For each of the Linked Type groups below, write "**T**" next to each symptom that you experience *at least once a month* **or each condition listed that has been diagnosed.** Write "**F**" next to each symptom or condition that does not apply to you.

Linked Type A

_____ Constipation (less than one bowel movement a day, or hard or firm stools that cause some straining)

_____ IBS/IBD, Gastritis, Ulcerative Colitis or Crohn's

_____ Frequent bad breath

_____ Extra weight in stomach area

_____ Acne around the mouth or chin

_____ Hemorrhoids

_____ Bloating, gas or intestinal discomfort after eating certain foods

_____ Very loose bowel movements after eating certain foods

_____ TOTAL TRUE

Linked Type B

_____ Nausea, and or sweating and or pain in upper abdomen after eating

_____ Gall stones or gall bladder removal

_____ Dry skin or dry hair

_____ High cholesterol or high triglyceride levels

_____ PMS symptoms and or heavy periods

_____ Joint pain

_____ Abdominal discomfort after eating fatty, greasy foods or red meat

_____ Bowel movements that occasionally or often float in the toilet bowl instead of sinking to the bottom of the toilet bowl

_____ TOTAL TRUE

Linked Type C

_____ Low or no appetite in the morning

_____ Irritable or lightheaded when hungry

_____ Iron-deficient anemia

_____ Nausea after taking supplements or after eating certain foods

_____ Heartburn, acid reflux or GERD
_____ High levels of stress
_____ Bouts of sadness or depression
_____ Either frequent craving of protein or an aversion/dislike to protein
_____ TOTAL TRUE

Linked Type D

_____ Vaginal yeast infections or toenail fungus
_____ Skin rashes of any kind (eczema, dermatitis, Rosacea)
_____ Sleep issues such as insomnia, bad dreams or up in the middle of the night
_____ Crave sugar or sugary foods
_____ Crave refine carbohydrates
_____ Irritable often for no apparent reason or mood swings
_____ Brain feels foggy or memory feels weak
_____ Trouble getting up in the morning
_____ TOTAL TRUE

2. Because the body works as a whole system and not independently of each internal system, it is normal to find several true symptoms in several different Linked Types, but one Linked Type should rise above the others. Count the number of true items for each Linked Type and write the corresponding total in each corresponding Total True blank. The section where you have the greatest number of True items is your dietary type.

    In the event of a tie between two or more Linked Type groups:

    a. Score each TRUE item in each group that tied according to how often you experience each symptom or condition using the number scale below:

        1 = once a month or less

        2 = more than once a month, but less than three times a week

        3 = three or more times a week or condition has been diagnosed

    b. Total the numeric values you indicated for each Linked Type group scored. The group with the highest total score is your true Linked Type.

3. Familiarize yourself with the corresponding Linked Type A, B, C or D food list, meal plan and recipes provided in this book as you continue to the next part of the book. Feel free to use other Linked Type Recipes with substitutions if necessary to fit your Linked Type Food List.

CHAPTER 4

AVOIDING COMMON MISTAKES

Even the most explicit dietary plans can be misinterpreted, and mistakes can be made. Unfortunately some of these mistakes may be the difference between success and failure. Mistakes can slow down progress or even result in weight gain. Your progress is only as good as your understanding of the plan itself and your commitment to it. This chapter gives you some helpful tips to keep you from making some common mistakes.

Water Intake

The number one rule of good health and fitness is to hydrate well. Water helps lubricate our joints, helps give us energy, helps keep our brain and blood healthy, helps flush fat and helps reduce inflammation. Most of us do not realize how important clean water is for the body. Failing to drink the proper amount of water is one of the most common mistakes people make.

How much is enough? Divide your body weight by two. The resulting number equals the number of fluid ounces of purified, filtered water you need to drink each day to be properly hydrated. *Do not exceed a gallon of water per day.* So for example, if your weight is over 300 lbs, then you will drink a maximum of one gallon of water (128 ounces) even though your weight divided by two equals 150. Do not forget to recalculate water intake as you lose significant weight.

The quality of your water is very important for both its purity and for when you need electrolytes. First, make sure it is clean and pure. Reverse osmosis or carbon-filtered waters are some of the best purified water, as is spring water that is bottled at a source that is not a municipal drinking source. Municipal drinking water is fancy for tap water. If you feel like you need to flavor your water, you can (as long as your choices fall in line with fruit and vegetable allowances in your Linked Type) use a slice or wedge of real lemon, lime, orange, strawberry or a few whole or halved small berries, cucumber slices or real mint leaves. All packaged or bottled juice, sports, or specialty drinks, including diet drinks, are not allowed while focusing on your weight and will compromise your progress and your health.

If you are exercising more than thirty minutes at a stretch and are over the age of thirteen, it is important to replenish electrolytes during exercise and after physical activity. We lose approximately two quarts of water per day through sweat from normal activity and urine. We will lose more during exercise or strenuous activity. You can weigh yourself on a scale before and after exercise to see how much water weight you have lost. This amount is crucial to replace directly following your exercise. Sports drinks are usually full of sugar, which means lots of unhealthy calories. If you really want to replenish the electrolytes, consume coconut water instead of sports drinks.

Believe it or not, the time of day that you drink water can make a big difference. The following pointers will help you benefit most from the water you drink by optimizing the time of the day it is consumed for the best results.

1. Drink a glass of water first thing in the morning on an empty stomach. Drinking first thing in the morning helps wake up the digestion system increasing optimal metabolic function.
2. Drink another glass of water two hours before bed. Drinking before bed helps flush toxins during the detoxification and rejuvenation of sleep. Since toxins are commonly stored in our fat, flushing toxins is like flushing fat.
3. Eating simply, as recommended in this program, helps rid the body of toxins more readily thus enhancing water's effect. For extra cleansing and fat flushing, squeeze half a fresh lemon into your morning and evening water. Lemon in water helps stimulate your metabolism and helps your liver function better. Your liver likes the help; it is your main filtering organ.
4. Drink a glass of water before reaching for a snack. Sometimes you are just thirsty and don't realize it. Rule out thirst first before reaching for food.
5. Another key moment you may confuse thirst and hunger is right after eating a meal that is heavy in *sodium chloride* (table salt). Too much table salt in a meal can increase your thirst. If you find yourself hungry within approximately thirty minutes after you finish eating, you are most likely thirsty, not hungry.

On a side note:

If at this time, you are especially hungry for something sweet after your meal, you most likely consumed too much grain, animal protein, or both resulting in the sugar cravings. In order to avoid the post-grain or post-animal-protein sugar cravings, keep your grain and animal protein portions the size of your fist.

Basically, your stomach is the size of your fist, and your body may struggle with proteins and grains. When you consume more than can fit into your stomach at one digestive sitting, your stomach enlarges causing metabolism to slow greatly and unwanted digestive symptoms to occur.

Because they can metabolize in under an hour, fruits and vegetables are different; there is no need for portion control. Portions of heavier, slower to digest foods, such as animal proteins and grains, should always remain the size of your fist or less, small enough to keep your stomach from enlarging.

Read Labels for Hidden Ingredients

Please read your labels very carefully. Many, many packaged foods will have unexpected ingredients. It is very easy to grab a chip, soup, nut butter, or other packaged food and make an assumption about what is inside the container. Even though whole, processed food will give you the fastest results, many of you will look for times when you can skirt around the preparation of a meal from scratch. So here are some common things to beware of:

1. Chips may contain vegetable oils that are not allowed on your plan.
2. Soups may contain gluten, dairy or vegetable oils that are not allowed on your plan.
3. Nut butter may contain sugar or oils that are not allowed on your plan.
4. Canned food may contain wheat, sugar, or oils. For example tuna packed in water can also contain other ingredients besides water, such as vegetable broth; tuna in olive oil may still contain soybean oil or canola oil. Only tunas found at a health food store or in the health food section of your grocery store are free of additives. It's best to avoid the general selection of canned tuna.
5. Always, always read your ingredient label on the back or side of the package, and never make the assumption of what the label says in the front.

Eat Breakfast

An absolutely fundamental rule to follow for optimal health and fitness is to make sure you always eat breakfast. A very common misconception is the belief that less is more, so you might start your day believing that completely skipping a meal is even better than eating a low-calorie meal. If you've been using a calorie-counting diet plan this can appear to make sense; eating no calories has to be better than eating less calories, right?

You might have used a cup of coffee for the energy you should have gotten from food to begin your day. Coffee gives us empty calories with false energy provided by caffeine. Your brain needs a significant number of good calories to function optimally, especially in the morning when, for most of us, a great deal of mental energy is necessary. Our brains and bodies need real, good calories to gain mental and physical energy. By the end of the day, if you did not get enough calories to support your mental *and* physical day, the body may demand more. Calories obtained after dark, especially late at night or right before bedtime, are less likely to be used by the body.

Sleep is supposed to be the time of rest and rejuvenation for the digestive system. If you wake up with undigested food in your system, you probably have little to no appetite first thing in the morning. But, you still need energy, so you reach for that coffee and start the cycle all over again. Break the cycle! Eat breakfast, especially a breakfast with protein! You need to get your body and brain going in the morning.

Avoid Late Night Eating

A cardinal rule of weight loss is to avoid eating after 9:00 pm. Avoiding food after dark is ideal, but we really get into digestive trouble after 9:00 pm. Late night binging is often the result of eating too little first thing in the morning or throughout the day. Eastern philosophy suggests that the digestive system runs in harmony with the sun. As morning approaches, the digestive system is ready to move from other tasks to digestion of foods. Digestion gets stronger at the break of day, is strongest around noon, and then slows down at dusk. By the time we are into absolute darkness of night, your body would much rather rest and recuperate through detoxification, instead of digesting another meal.

Your body is especially not interested in digesting junk food or dessert late at night either. If avoiding late night eating is a real struggle for you, begin slowly by eating a plain fruit allowed by your Linked Type. When you are ready, give up the fruit for chamomile tea, and eventually eliminate everything except water.

Eat with the Sun

If you take into consideration the philosophy that your digestion runs in harmony with the sun, then you can also run your consumption along a similar train of thought. Upon sunrise, your digestion is beginning to wake up. Wake it up gently by eating a light pre-breakfast such as lemon water and fruit or vegetable. Then, about thirty minutes later, move to medium breakfast. By noon your digestion is in full force. Eat your largest meal of the day at lunch (between 11:00 am and 1:00 pm). By sunset, your digestion is slowing down again, so you then want to eat your smallest meal at dinner. The saying "Eat breakfast like a king, lunch like a prince and dinner like a pauper" is based on a similar notion.

Avoid Television Eating and Eating in Bed

A fundamental rule of this program is no eating in front of the television. Period. When we eat in front of the television, we lose all connection with the celebration and appreciation of what we are eating. As a result, we often rush through the meal with very little conscious thought and are more likely to overeat. Don't eat in bed either. The bed is a sacred place of sleep and, if applicable, intimacy with your partner. It is not a sacred space for food. The only place you should eat is at the table with gratitude and appreciation, with good conversation or, if you eat alone, reflective silence.

Avoid Alcohol

Another important consideration is to avoid alcohol while working on your weight or other health goals. Wine, beer and hard liquor are all very relaxing and slow metabolism down. When you are trying to lose weight the goal is to keep your metabolism as active and stimulated as possible. Whole, unprocessed, unadulterated foods are easiest for the body to metabolize. If you relax at the end of your day with a glass of wine or other form of alcohol, then the next two chapters will give you some ideas on how to relax in a more constructive manner while pursuing the Linked Diet.

Snack on Apples

One of the greatest challenges while dieting is snacking. This is a tremendous area of weakness and temptation for most of us. Instead of letting the snack monster rule you, you can rule the snack monster by eating three apples every day. First of all, if you can find three times to eat an apple in a single day, you will find yourself eating very few snacks; cravings will be much more manageable. Apples help curb your appetite and provide good soluble and insoluble fiber, which is great for digestion and metabolism. Apples help fight allergies, help clean your teeth, and help fight against cancer. The list of benefits from a single apple is very long, hence the phrase "An apple a day keeps the doctor away." Mostly, apples help you manage cravings and aid digestion and metabolism.

Control Sugar and Carb Cravings

Remember the effect of grain and animal protein portions. If your sugar cravings come about thirty minutes after your meal, then you had too much grain or animal protein at that meal. Limit portions to half the size of your fist or less. However, if you find your refined carbohydrate or sugar cravings do not fall within that time window and are unbearable, even with the apples, then try these tips.

1. Consume a small amount of non-animal protein (such as almonds or cashews) when the cravings first strike. This is actually the true need of your body when you are craving refined carbohydrates or sugar. The body actually wants the feel-good chemicals that are supplied through amino acids, which are proteins broken down in the body. Because our taste palate has been altered by a poor diet, you may think you want the quick fix of refined carbs or sugar rather than the true solution: protein. A handful of roasted almonds could very well do the trick!

2. If eating protein does not relieve the cravings, try adding a 500-mg-dose, once a day of the supplement L-glutamine (an amino acid that helps control cravings). Increase to 1,000 mg if you find the low dose does not control the cravings. You should exercise caution with L-glutamine, and use for only one to three months and with your doctor's permission if you take prescription medications to avoid any contraindications with your medications. Just remember that every time you eat too many sugars or refined carbohydrates, you may interfere in your body's ability to absorb proteins efficiently, which further reduces weight loss success by increasing sugar and carb cravings.

Avoid Oil Mistakes

Most of you will change the kind of fat you use while on a good weight plan. The problem with changing your oil is that all oils are not the same. The biggest difference is their tolerance to heat. If you make the switch to olive oil, make sure to use only extra-virgin olive oil. Other olive oils are not a healthy olive oil. You must avoid heating olive oil at high temperatures. It breaks down in high heat and is no longer nutritionally valuable. Instead, heat olive oil on low to medium temperatures or avoid heating it altogether. Coconut oil withstands high heat better, and is the better alternative for roasting or baking.

Coconut oil is a saturated fat, but it is not an inflammatory saturated fat. In fact, coconut oil contains medium-chain triglycerides that may improve fat oxidation and stimulate metabolic energy. However, it is very high in calories and contains lauric acid, which can help the body balance weight by stimulating metabolism or by helping someone gain weight if that is needed. It should be used with caution and in moderation. Therefore, it is best for roasting and baking, not pan-frying or sautéing. Organic butter, if allowed by your Linked Type, is another option for high heat cooking.

Accountability with a Buddy

A strong commitment to your overall health is just as important as the food you eat as well as your thoughts and actions. A strong commitment is not only a promise to yourself, but a way to hold yourself accountable. Many of us are challenged to hold ourselves accountable and could use a buddy to help us in this area. If you feel you are inclined to cut corners, have cheat days, lie about what you are eating, or fight with yourself to stay on the plan, then you need to seek a professional that will support you.

Always avoid using your spouse or someone you are romantically involved with as this is an unhealthy dynamic in your intimate relationships. Choose someone who will do this diet with you, or find a professional who will support this process. Let this person know what you are doing. Ask if you can send a copy of your food diary and report what you are eating on a weekly basis. Just this simple act of having to report to someone other than yourself can help keep you on track. If you feel a smart phone app is enough, then use an app with caution, since it does not provide the same kind of accountability as a professional. The clients in my office on an accountability plan do much better than those completely on their own.

Turbo Charged

If you want to increase the speed with which you see results, accelerate your progress by giving up solid foods one or two meals a day or for one 24-hour period each week. The digestion of solid foods is a slower more involved process in the body, whereas liquid foods are easier to digest and stimulate the metabolism. Instead of solid foods, consume either fresh, homemade juices (such as carrot, apple and beet) or consume homemade vegetable or meat broth.

Some of you will find the raw juice will be a little irritating to your system, and should consume the broth. Or on colder days, the raw juice may not seem as appealing. Anytime the body is given a break from solid foods, if done in moderation, the digestive system is given a chance to rest. As we know from being sick with a cold or flu, rest is imperative to our recovery. The different systems in our body are no different, a bit of rest goes a long way toward healing.

This elimination of solid foods is called fasting. Fasting beyond one day per week should be exercised with caution, and should ultimately be supervised by a healthcare professional that has experience with detoxification and fasting protocols.

Additional Testing

Consider several different kinds of functional testing to see how your bodily systems are working in relationship to food and stress. One type of functional test is a comprehensive digestive stool analysis. Another is a hormone panel and another is a thyroid panel. Most doctors can test your thyroid and or hormones, but a digestive stool analysis can be done through my office or with practitioners that have functional testing as part of their services offered. A comprehensive stool analysis requires the collection of one to three days of your bowel movements in the privacy of your home. This test looks for good and bad bacteria, your levels of nutrient absorption, any infectious agents and other small details that demonstrate how your body handles food. A digestive stool analysis may reveal any bacterial infection in your gut that may be one reason you have difficulty reaching your weight loss goals. If your hormones are off, you may have slower weight loss results. Or lastly, a thyroid imbalance may also slow weight loss results.

When thyroid testing is ordered consider the following: Some doctors only check your thyroid-stimulating hormone (TSH) level when you ask for your thyroid to be tested. Some will go so far as to test TSH and free T4 (*thyroxine*) levels, but anyone who has had weight issues for longer than 5 years, is over the age of 35, and considers their stress level high should get the full panel of TSH, free T4, free T3 (*triiodothyronine*) and thyroid antibody levels.

Conclusion

Hopefully these tips will help you avoid some common mistakes and guide you through common struggles that occur when changing your diet. Keeping yourself accountable and keeping a positive attitude are also very important pieces of your plan. The next chapter provides you with a series of daily, mental exercises to help you stay focused and address some underlying mental and emotional issues that may be keeping you from losing the weight and keeping it off.

CHAPTER 5

GETTING STARTED: MINDSET STEPS

Much of the stress we face is caused by our own personal perceptions. When your perceptions hinder your progress toward a very important goal, it might be time to look at those perceptions and even go so far as to redefine them. In my experience, many weight loss clients give up on their dietary plan because of their perceptions of themselves and the world around them. These perceptions are significant to their failure. Your perceptions—positive and/or negative—will have a significant impact on your success.

If you never change your thinking, you will never change your actions. Remember that what we think, we become. So believing in ourselves as beautiful and worthy of a healthy and fit body is just as important as actually eating certain foods. If you only think about what you *cannot* eat, then it is your thinking that will keep you from moving to a place of success. If you fulfill your dietary requirements, but all the while you are dreaming of the time when you can eat those foods again, you are undermining your own success. In fact, with those thoughts, you are making a subconscious plan to put the weight back on even before you lose it. Focusing on what you *cannot* eat gives you a victim perception of your diet experience. Victim mentality is typically not associated with success. If your goal is to be successful with weight loss and true fitness, then you have to leave the victim mentality behind.

The first step is to change your opinion of eating and food itself. You have to look at your perception of food. Do you associate healthy food with the punishment of being on a diet? Is unhealthy food associated with such feelings as celebration, reward, stress relief, and even intimacy? We live in a culture that promotes a number of these mentalities. "Let's go for ice cream!" may be heard after the team wins their game or when we want to do something special with another person. We might go out for a specialty coffee to feel good about ourselves, as if a high-calorie, fancy coffee drink holds more status than an ordinary cup of coffee. If we already view ourselves in a negative light, then we may seek anything that helps us think we feel okay with ourselves. We elevate ordinary food experiences in such a way that transforms our perception of ourselves and often allows these unhealthy foods to make us feel special.

The reality is you are special no matter what you eat. It may sound trite, but you are special because you are a unique person inside regardless of what your outward appearance may be. Unfortunately, we live in a society that views the outside as more important than the inside. This is compounded with the capitalistic culture that tells us to adorn the body with clothes, jewelry, makeup and other beauty treatments for just the right look, further accentuating the focus on the outside. We have to understand that food, especially unhealthy food, does not make us special. In fact, these unhealthy foods may even change our moods, emotions and behaviors and cause us to be less special on the inside. At the end of the day, we are what we eat. And if what we think, what we feel and what we do is the product of what we are, then what we think, feel and do is the product of what we eat.

There is also another consideration that you may not want to even consider, much less admit. As painful as it may be, it is important to consider whether or not you secretly, or even unconsciously, gain benefit from being overweight. You may have just reacted to reading that statement and think "No way!" But please keep reading. All things—even negative things have a benefit to us, we just may not consciously realize the benefits. After all, the possible consequences of many negative things are usually enough to outweigh any consideration of a possible benefit. But behavior patterns, both positive and negative, that become habitual are giving us some benefit, usually something intangible. Part of the powerful ability to make a change in our lives in any area is to admit the negative *and* positive reasons we do what we do. Then, we can be more honest with ourselves about what we really want to change—weight and overall health in this case. Admitting there is a benefit to overeating or eating certain unhealthy food allows us to make changes that link the benefits to being fit.

Typically, the needs we are trying to meet with food are either emotional, physical or both. The times we eat out of physical need are important and should be filled with good choices to help us be the best version of our physical self. The times we eat for emotional reasons are equally important. Keep in mind, when we eat poor food choices for emotional reasons, we are trying to meet a real need in a destructive manner instead of a constructive manner. Emotional eating for someone who is overweight and trying to lose the weight is destructive. Many individuals give up on their diets before reaching their goals when any emotional void that used to be filled by unhealthy food has been ignored for far too long. *The most powerful work you can do for yourself is to stay committed mentally until you get the results you want.*

You will need to find new ways to fill emotional needs. When you embrace a different way of thinking about food and find better ways to fill emotional needs you will be embracing not just a diet or weight loss plan, but a life plan. Good, healthy eating can be a permanent and lifelong commitment.

All of this may seem like a tall order. This chapter aims to help you reset your thought patterns, solidify what you are learning about your individual food needs, and change your eating patterns to be in line with your new mindset. You will do so by completing a series of exercises as assigned to each day for seven consecutive days. Each day has one or more exercises to be completed on the specified day. You may use an empty notebook if you would like more room. These exercises are as equally important to your success as following your food recommendations. *This is where the mental and emotional work supports the work at the table and in the gym.* This is where you take care of the inside as well as the outside. This is where you address the missing link between your thoughts and actions while losing the weight.

Mindset Steps: Day 1

Exercise 1.1

Write down at least seven foods that you used to believe you should eat to be more fit and healthy. Next to each food you identified write down how often you used to eat this particular food.

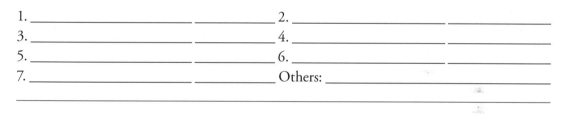

1. _____ _____ 2. _____ _____
3. _____ _____ 4. _____ _____
5. _____ _____ 6. _____ _____
7. _____ _____ Others: _____
_____

Any surprises? Do you eat more or less of a particular food than you expected? In either scenario, actually writing out the top foods you used to think you should eat helps brings awareness to how different your thinking is on the Linked Diet.

Exercise 1.2

Expressing our gratitude reminds us of the big picture, which helps prevent getting caught up in the small stresses and minutia that keep us from being able to rise above challenges of our day to day life. When we have a big picture focus and we rise above the challenges, we are less likely to choose foods that will not help us be our best selves and more likely to live in such a way that totally supports our big picture. Write down three sentences about what you are most grateful for.

_____
_____
_____

Exercise 1.3

Begin keeping a food diary of what you eat. Write down portions in terms of cups, handfuls and fist sizes or food items themselves. Do not count calories or grams. For example, 1 c of fruit salad, 1 c of salad, ½ c or two handfuls of raw almonds, 1 piece of wild Alaskan salmon half the size of my fist, 1 hardboiled egg, 1 apple,, etc.

It is good to keep track of your day. You need to make note of the positive and negative food choices you made. Remember your Linked Diet Food List specifies which foods should make up 60–80% of your diet and which foods should make up 20–40% and less of the food you eat. Keeping a food diary helps keep you accountable. We will talk more about accountability in the next chapter. For now, it is important to keep the food diary each day.

Breakfast: _____

Snack: _____

Lunch: _____

Dinner: _____

Snack: _____

Drinks:_____

Water Intake: _____

Mindset Steps: Day 2

Exercise 2.1

Write down at least ten positive characteristics of yourself. The easier it is for you to articulate negative characteristics, both in yourself and the people you are closest to, the harder it may seem to identify the positive. And that is exactly why, it is so important to make the effort and take the time necessary to write out your positive characteristics. You need to remember how wonderful you truly are. Don't stop at 1, 3, 7 or even 9. Go ahead and list at least 10. If it helps, list those positive things you think no one notices. Those things count too!

10 characteristics that make me wonderful are…

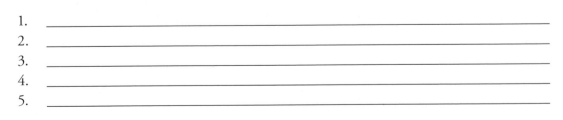

1. _____
2. _____
3. _____
4. _____
5. _____

6. _____

7. _____

8. _____

9. _____

10. _____

You may believe that everyone sees your weight first in everything you do. The truth is that most of the time it is you who sees it first—not others. You are so much more than your weight. For each characteristic above, write down how your weight gets in the way of this positive characteristic manifesting itself on a regular basis. This is key to understanding that you are not your weight, but your weight may very well be interfering in you being the best version of yourself you can be.

My weight hinders my best characteristics by…

Characteristic 1. _____

Characteristic 2. _____

Characteristic 3. _____

Characteristic 4. _____

Characteristic 5. _____

Characteristic 6 _____

Characteristic 7. _____

Characteristic 8. _____

Characteristic 9. _____

Characteristic 10. _____

Exercise 2.2

Speak your gratitude and identify what you feel went well today. Continue to write down three to five sentences about what you are grateful for. In addition, write down ten things you did well today. Yes, you do have a list of things that you did well today. Stretch the truth if you have to. Putting a positive spin on the plain things that happened in our day helps us think positively about ourselves. These can be little things or big things or a combination. It is only when we can shift our perception from the negative that we can stay motivated.

I am grateful for…

_____

_____

_____

_____

_____

_____

10 Things I Did Well Today

1. _____
2. _____
3. _____
4. _____
5. _____
6. _____
7. _____
8. _____
9. _____
10. _____

Exercise 2.3

Keep your food diary.

Breakfast: _____

Snack: _____

Lunch: _____

Dinner: _____

Snack: _____

Drinks:_____

Water Intake: _____

Mindset Steps: DAY 3

Exercise 3.1

Write down all the reasons you eat. Take time to really think about this one because, when we eat beyond our daily physical needs, we might be eating rather thoughtlessly.

Thoughtless eating might look like this: It's been a hard day at work; you leave stressed and tired and pull into a drive through thinking, "Right now I am exhausted from a stressful day at work, and I am here because I deserve it." It is true we are stressed. You did work hard and you are tired, but is bad food really the answer? Or the reward you want? If you identify all the reasons you eat you will bring those reasons to the front of your thinking. For many of us, emotionally eating is triggered by stress, reward, boredom, loneliness, and social pressures. But underneath these reasons are deeper, hidden reasons, so *be very specific*. If you eat when you have a bad day at work, this is more than just writing down the word stress. You might need to write down "I eat after a stressful day at work because I am afraid of standing up to my boss." Your emotional need may then be letting go of fear and building up courage.

For each emotional need you identify, try to come up with an alternative way to fulfill the emotional need other than eating. For example, you could write down "At the end of a stressful day, I will take a hot bath." You may not be able to come up with these alternative reasons on the first go, so feel free to leave it and come back to it another day. Remember, the reasons we eat are still present; and when we change our eating, we still have to create alternative solutions to fill the emotional need we were trying to meet when we overate.

Emotional Need	Alternative Strategy

Exercise 3.2

Express gratitude, what you did well today, and articulate better ways to problem solve or feel better about a situation.

I am grateful for…

_____

_____

_____

_____

_____

10 Things I Did Well Today

1. _____
2. _____
3. _____
4. _____
5. _____
6. _____
7. _____
8. _____
9. _____
10. _____

Pick one alternative strategy from Exercise 3.1 that you will try to do over the next week instead of emotional eating.

Write your new strategy here:

_____

_____

Going forward, you can use this new kind of thinking as a tool throughout your days. When you feel the temptation to eat for emotional reasons, remind yourself the first step is to make a different choice. Stop and ask yourself "Am I eating for a physical reason or an emotional reason?" If the reason is physical and you are about to make an unhealthy choice, stop and ask yourself "Can I make a different choice?" If the reason is emotional and you are reaching for food to make yourself feel better, stop and ask yourself, "Can I do something different instead of eat?"

Exercise 3.3

Keep your food diary of the day.

Breakfast: _____

Snack: _____

Lunch: _____

Dinner: _____

Snack: _____

Drinks:_____

Water Intake: _____

Mindset Steps: DAY 4

Exercise 4.1

Write down the people, places and experiences that make you feel good about yourself. This list is a magical tapestry in the uniqueness of you. These are great reasons for you to be committed to your plan. You may have your career on that list, or maybe your son or daughter, or your sister. Maybe it's your church. Maybe your best friend or the trip you took to the beach last summer. Be very specific in your list. Savor this list; and when you feel discouraged or are having a particularly rough day, come back to this list for encouragement.

People that make me feel good about myself are…

_____

_____

_____

Places that make me feel good about myself are…

_____

_____

_____

Experiences that make me feel good about myself are…

Exercise 4.2

Write down three to five sentences about what you are grateful for and ten things that you did well today.

I am grateful for…

10 Things I Did Well Today

1. _____
2. _____
3. _____
4. _____
5. _____
6. _____
7. _____
8. _____
9. _____
10. _____

Exercise 4.3

Keep your food diary of the day.

Breakfast: _____
Snack: _____
Lunch: _____
Dinner: _____
Snack: _____
Drinks: _____
Water Intake: _____

Mindset Steps: DAY 5

Exercise 5.1

Choose a role model. Write down the name of someone who you can consider a role model. If you don't already consider this person a role model, this may be a completely foreign idea, and you will have to spend some time selecting one. Make sure you list at least ten reasons why this person is a role model. *None of those reasons can be that person's weight or physical appearance.* It is so easy to get caught up in the superficial image based on the culture we live in that promotes youth and thin bodies. Successful thinking is about weight loss as a means to an end so that you can be a healthier version of yourself. If you are trying to emulate the cultural images of what is healthy, you may lose motivation and give up on yourself. A good role model is someone who you can admire because of qualities that have nothing to do with their weight.

Name _____

10 Reasons He/She Is a Role Model

1. _____
2. _____
3. _____
4. _____
5. _____
6. _____
7. _____
8. _____
9. _____
10. _____

A good role model is important to help you stay motivated. When you are down and thinking you might give up, think about what your role model might do in the very same scenario.

Exercise 5.2

Write down three to five sentences about what you are grateful for and write down ten things that you did well today.

I am grateful for…

_____
_____
_____
_____
_____
_____

10 Things I Did Well Today

1. _____
2. _____
3. _____

4. _____

5. _____

6. _____

7. _____

8. _____

9. _____

10. _____

Exercise 5.3

Keep your food diary.

Breakfast: _____

Snack: _____

Lunch: _____

Dinner: _____

Snack: _____

Drinks:_____

Water Intake: _____

Mindset Steps: DAY 6

Exercise 6.1

You should now be a few days into the program and following your food recommendations. The first few days can present a lot of cravings, or you may be tempted to focus on the struggle instead of the goodness of your plan.

Make a list of foods you find very appealing and healthy. You will need to use this list during tomorrow's exercise of making a meal plan for the following week; but for today, just make a list of foods you have tried and liked or foods you would like to try. After you have made your list, rate each food. Give up to four stars based on what you believe is the best on your list.

_____

_____

_____

_____

_____

_____
_____
_____
_____
_____
_____
_____

Exercise 6.2

Write down three to five gratitude statements and ten things that went well today.
I am grateful for…

_____
_____
_____
_____
_____
_____

10 Things I Did Well Today

1. _____
2. _____
3. _____
4. _____
5. _____
6. _____
7. _____
8. _____
9. _____
10. _____

Exercise 6.3

Keep your food diary for the day.

Breakfast: _____

Snack: _____

Lunch: _____

Dinner: _____

Snack: _____

Drinks:_____

Water Intake: _____

Mindset Steps: DAY 7

Exercise 7.1

Make a weekly meal plan and grocery list for the upcoming week. First, examine your first week's food diary. Identify where your strengths are to be commended and where your weaknesses need to be strengthened. Make a formal decision to make a new plan for the upcoming week and take one more step to better eating for better health. If you followed your Linked Type meal plan at the back of the book, now is a great time to sit and see how well you can do on your own. Using your Linked Type meal plan as a guide, see if you can create some of your own meals and learn to use your food list by yourself.

If the thought of a creating a whole new meal plan based on your Linked Type food list is overwhelming at this point, use your Linked Type meal plan as-is with the exception of two or three meals that you pick to vary. Write down how you will vary the meal plan and create your grocery list. Each week you can build up to creating your own complete meal plan by varying one or two more meals as you feel comfortable.

Week Two Meal Plan
Day 1:

Breakfast:_____

Lunch: _____

Snack: _____

Dinner: _____

Laura Kopec

Day 2:

Breakfast: _____

Lunch: _____

Snack: _____

Dinner: _____

Day 3:

Breakfast: _____

Lunch: _____

Snack: _____

Dinner: _____

Day 4:

Breakfast: _____

Lunch: _____

Snack: _____

Dinner: _____

Day 5:

Breakfast: _____

Lunch: _____

Snack: _____

Dinner: _____

Day 6:

Breakfast: _____

Lunch: _____

Snack: _____

Dinner: _____

Day 7:

Breakfast: _____
Lunch: _____
Snack: _____
Dinner: _____

Grocery List:

_____
_____
_____
_____
_____
_____
_____

Exercise 7.2

Write down three to five things you are grateful for and ten things that you did well today.
I am grateful for…

_____
_____
_____
_____
_____
_____

10 Things I Did Well Today

1. _____
2. _____
3. _____
4. _____
5. _____
6. _____
7. _____

8. _____
9. _____
10. _____

Exercise 7.3

Keep your food diary.

Breakfast: _____
Snack: _____
Lunch: _____
Dinner: _____
Snack: _____
Drinks:_____
Water Intake: _____

Way to go! You have completed the first week of the Linked Diet. It will get easier as you continue to tap into the strength of each link in your weight loss chain. Next, we take action steps to help support our new mindset and continue to build our new eating habits.

CHAPTER 6

GREAT START! ACTION STEPS TO KEEP GOING

Life is full of stress and complexities, challenges and blessings. In fact, it is the very fact that life is so full of complexities and challenges that we are having a fully human and enriched life, but we forget that. It seems so much easier to crave a dull life or escape our own lives in front of the television set, watching TV characters handle life, than to reach out and face our own challenges. But when we meet our challenges head on, we cannot deny it is a tremendous opportunity to grow and show ourselves—and the world around us—how we deal with those challenges positively.

If overeating was a coping strategy for life's stress and your diet feels like stress, then how will you ultimately succeed at your health and weight goals? You move away from eating as a stress response and toward eating healthily despite stress. You want to make sure that, while following your Linked Diet food recommendations, you are not overwhelmed by the commitment to your plan. In order to do this, it is important to understand exactly what is important to you and how to reach your weight loss goals.

Very likely, the action step exercises in this chapter were significant missing links of previous dieting attempts, especially if you did not see results or if you saw initial results but put the weight back on. These exercises are designed to help you continue to avoid unhealthy or emotional eating and build your dietary changes into lifestyle changes. *Please review all the exercises in advance; so that, if any call for advance planning, you are prepared.* Complete each of these exercises on the specified day of your Linked Diet. You can continue to use a notebook if you need additional space.

Action Steps: DAY 8

Exercise 8.1

Create an emergency kit for your car. Gather items today, if possible.

This kind of kit has been such a blessing to many of my clients. It kept them from throwing in the towel on numerous occasions. While dieting or living a healthier lifestyle, you will inevitably find yourself in a stressful scenario where you have no healthy food available to you. For example, your meeting at work ran over time, you missed lunch and now you are late to pick up the kids. Prior to your commitment to your health, you may have pulled into a drive-thru on the way to get the kids, but the drive-thru is not an option for you now that you have a new mindset. You are stressed, and you still need to eat. With an emergency kit, instead of going to the drive-thru, you can reach into your kit and pull out your raw almonds and water bottle, and you can tie yourself over until you get home.

Your emergency kit is not just about healthy snacks. Here's another scenario. You leave work early and plan to sit and wait for the kids at school. Normally, you might have stopped and indulged in an afternoon specialty coffee or a candy bar to unwind. You tell yourself, "I had a hard day, and I deserve a treat." Instead, you are going to reach into your emergency kit and get out a magazine or a novel, and you are going to unwind with a low stress book or magazine instead of eating. And you are going to tell yourself, "I had a hard day, but I am committed to my health and my plan, and I will not let my day run my life. I run my life." Let this become your mantra, "I run my life; my life does not run me."

Your emergency kit can be filled with other items to help with stress or boredom or some of the other mental and emotional reasons you used to eat. Make this kit as personal and inviting as you possibly can, and remember how special and unique you are while putting it together. Examples of items to go into your kit: water bottle (sometimes we are just thirsty and think we are hungry instead), trail mix or nuts, dried fruit, magazine, low-stress novel, small notebook for writing down thoughts, small Bible, crossword puzzle or other brain stimulation items. Good luck and have fun!

I gathered items for my emergency kit on this date: _____

Items in my emergency kit: _____

_____

_____

_____

_____

_____

_____

_____

_____

_____

_____

_____

Exercise 8.2

Write down three to five things you are grateful for and ten things that you did well today. Hopefully, you can add your completed emergency kit to your list of things done well.

I am grateful for...

_____
_____
_____
_____
_____
_____

10 Things I Did Well Today

1. _____
2. _____
3. _____
4. _____
5. _____
6. _____
7. _____
8. _____
9. _____
10. _____

Exercise 8.3

Keep your food diary.

Breakfast:_____
Snack: _____
Lunch: _____
Dinner: _____
Snack: _____
Drinks:_____
Water Intake: _____

Action Steps: DAY 9

Exercise 9.1

Create a space in your home just for you that will be a special and private place you can go without the temptations of food.

This may be a little bit more challenging, but the ultimate goal is to have a place to go to when you feel the at-home pressure of eating. It does not have to be a big area, and it can be an area that you already have in your home, but now you will think about it differently. Some examples are your bathtub, your bed, or a chair in your bedroom. Say aloud that this is your special place where you will come when you feel the temptation to cheat. Promise yourself to never bring food into this designated place.

After you have designated the spot and made your promise, place something there to remind you of its specialness like a candle, your notebook, or a personal item. Go to this spot when you used to eat out of boredom or stress. It is even better if you have a designated activity for the space. Here are some scenarios of your space that work for your good:

1. Your special space is your bathtub. You planned to do some work or some laundry after getting the kids to bed. Instead, you find yourself too tired and would usually decide to sit in front of the television, probably with some food that you cannot have anymore, to unwind. Instead, you decide to take those thirty minutes that you would have spent in front of the television, and you go take a hot bath.

2. You're special space is in your bedroom. You and a co-worker got into it at work today. All you can think about is unwinding in front of the television with a glass of wine or some ice cream. This is not a healthy way to unwind, and you have different priorities now that you are committed to your plan. Instead of drinking or eating, you are going to sit in your chair in your bedroom and read the really good book you started last year but never finished. Or you decide to write in your journal and focus on what you are grateful for and what you did right today.

Write a reflection about your new special place, how you plan to use it and what it will mean to you in this journey.

_____

_____

_____

_____

_____

_____
_____
_____
_____
_____
_____
_____
_____
_____
_____
_____
_____
_____
_____
_____
_____
_____
_____
_____
_____
_____
_____
_____
_____
_____
_____

Exercise 9.2

Write down three to five things you are grateful for and ten things that you did well today.
I am grateful for…

_____
_____
_____
_____
_____
_____

10 Things I Did Well Today

1. _____
2. _____
3. _____
4. _____
5. _____
6. _____
7. _____
8. _____
9. _____
10. _____

Exercise 9.3

Keep your food diary.

Breakfast: _____
Snack: _____
Lunch: _____
Dinner: _____
Snack: _____
Drinks: _____
Water Intake: _____

Action Steps: DAY 10

Exercise 10.1

What areas of your life are most important to you? Is it your children? Your spouse? Your career? Is it your leisure time? There are no right or wrong answers to this question. What is important to us is unique to each one of us and helps keep the world a magical place of individuality. Write down a list of the three most important areas of your life. Under each one of these, write three examples of how being healthier would benefit these areas. For example, if your spouse falls into your top three priorities, then you would write down reasons such as 1) being a better version of myself allows me to be more sexually interested and allows me to feel sexier with my spouse, 2) being a better version of myself means I have more energy to go on a date night at the end of the week, 3) being a better version of myself means I will not be afraid to have my picture taken with my spouse or my children.

The 3 Most Important Areas of My Life

1. _____

Ways being healthy will benefit this area: _

_____
_____
_____
_____

2. _____

Ways being healthy will benefit this area:

_____
_____
_____
_____

3. _____

Ways being healthy will benefit this area:

_____
_____
_____
_____
_____

Exercise 10.2

In addition to your gratitude list and list of things that you did well today, you will create three positive, present-tense affirmations to be used daily.

I am grateful for...

_____
_____
_____
_____

10 Things I Did Well Today

1. _____
2. _____
3. _____
4. _____
5. _____
6. _____
7. _____
8. _____
9. _____
10. _____

Next, write three positive, present-tense affirmations about you that reflect the future manifestation of the healthier version of you. Even if you have not actually achieved these goals, the idea is to turn wishful thinking into reachable and present parts of ourselves.

For example:

"I am healthy, and I am the weight I want to be."

"I have more energy."

"I am able to climb stairs without getting out of breath."

Daily Positive Affirmations

1. _____
_____

2. _____
_____

3. _____
_____

Exercise 10.3

Keep your food diary.

Breakfast: _____
Snack: _____
Lunch: _____
Dinner: _____

Snack: _____

Drinks:_____

Water Intake: _____

Action Steps: DAY 11

Exercise 11.1

Dream a little about how life will be different after reaching your goals. Most successful people had a very clear vision of the area in which they wanted to be successful. Having a healthy and fit body is not very different from choosing to be successful in another area. You have to decide to be successful, and you have to envision what life will be like once you achieve the success. There is great power in writing down this vision. We move positive thinking from the recesses of our subconscious minds into the forefront of our thinking when we write it down. Then our actions are more likely to become linked to our goals.

Long-lasting weight loss is not just about changing your outside, but about making healthy choices that will help you realize other goals as well. So, instead of just dreaming of the new body image you want to have, you need to actually write down all the new ways your health goals will improve and enhance your life.

My Life after Losing Weight

_____

_____

_____

_____

_____

_____

_____

_____

_____

_____

_____

_____

_____

_____

_____

_____

_____
_____
_____
_____
_____
_____
_____
_____
_____
_____
_____

Exercise 11.2

Write your gratitude entry, ten things that you did well today, and your daily present-tense, positive affirmations.

I am grateful for…

_____
_____
_____
_____
_____
_____

10 Things I Did Well Today

1. _____
2. _____
3. _____
4. _____
5. _____
6. _____
7. _____
8. _____
9. _____
10. _____

Daily Positive Affirmations:

1. _____
   _____

2. _____
   _____

3. _____
   _____

Exercise 11.3

Keep your food diary.

Breakfast: _____
Snack: _____
Lunch: _____
Dinner: _____
Snack: _____
Drinks:_____
Water Intake: _____

Action Steps: DAY 12

Exercise 12.1

Write down a list of areas you *believe* you have to be perfect in.

_____
_____
_____

Perfection is unattainable, and the desire to be perfect is unhealthy. Too many of us with eating issues also have perfection issues. Thus, a heavy cloud constantly overshadows any success we are experiencing by dripping drops of perceived failure for not having the perfect body. Or maybe our perfectionism is so strong that the cloud floods us with the desire to give up on our eating before we even try to be committed to a plan.

To be perfect means we can only feel defeated by our failures, instead of feeling encouraged by learning from our mistakes. Release yourself of the quest for perfection and give yourself permission to make mistakes. When you give yourself permission to make mistakes and get back on the horse, you can be okay with the ups and down of weight loss. If you make a mistake while on the Linked Diet, think of it as an opportunity to learn—not as a failure or a reason to give up. Our mistakes, our challenges, and our path can be a chance to grow and learn positively only if we choose to do so. It is only through growing out of the negative and learning to grow into the positive that we truly get to be better versions of ourselves.

For each area in which you believe you have to be perfect, write down what you think would happen if you made a mistake in that area. Then, put a line through it and write down what would really happen if you made a mistake.

For example:

- Area of Perfection is "I have to be a perfect daughter."
- Result of making a mistake might be "If I am not a perfect daughter, my mother will not talk to me."
- Correction: "~~If I am not a perfect daughter, my mother will not talk to me.~~ This is not true of any healthy mother. My mother does not expect perfection. If she does that is her issue, not mine. If I make a mistake, she will likely criticize me, but she won't stop talking to me altogether. Can I live with her criticism? YES! I won't like it, but I can live with it."

Laura Kopec

_____
_____
_____
_____
_____
_____
_____

Exercise 12.2

Write your gratitude entry, the ten things that you did well today, and your daily present-tense, positive affirmations.

I am grateful for…

_____
_____
_____
_____
_____
_____

10 Things I Did Well Today

1. _____
2. _____
3. _____
4. _____
5. _____
6. _____
7. _____
8. _____
9. _____
10. _____

Daily Positive Affirmations:

1. _____
_____

2. _____
   _____

3. _____
   _____

Exercise 12.3

Keep your food diary.

Breakfast: _____
Snack: _____
Lunch: _____
Dinner: _____
Snack: _____
Drinks:_____
Water Intake: _____

Action Steps: DAY 13

Exercise 13.1

Write a letter to your overweight self. Sometimes we carry guilt inside our bodies, and this guilt needs to be freed. Sometimes we need to forgive ourselves of the path we have taken in order to leave that path behind. Speak freely to your overweight self whether you need to tell her she is okay, or that she has always tried, or that you understand how hard it has been to deal with the challenges of her life. Whatever you write to yourself, it is necessary and will free you from more negative self-talk. You can write this letter on your computer, or you can write it here or in your notebook where you can reflect upon it at a later time.

Dear _____,

_____
_____
_____
_____
_____
_____
_____

_____
_____
_____
_____
_____
_____
_____
_____
_____
_____
_____
_____

Exercise 13.2

Write your gratitude entry, the ten things that went well today and your daily present-tense, positive affirmations.

I am grateful for…

_____
_____
_____
_____
_____
_____

10 Things I Did Well Today

1. _____
2. _____
3. _____
4. _____
5. _____
6. _____
7. _____
8. _____
9. _____
10. _____

Daily Positive Affirmations:

1. _____

   _____

2. _____

   _____

3. _____

   _____

Exercise 13.3

Keep your food diary.

Breakfast: _____
Snack: _____
Lunch: _____
Dinner: _____
Snack: _____
Drinks:_____
Water Intake: _____

Action Steps: DAY 14

Exercise 14.1

Make a healthy meal for a friend. A big part of eating in our culture is socialization. When we are on a diet, we have a tendency to apologize for the diet or for not being able to participate in unhealthy food choices. We say things like, "I can't have that right now, I'm on a diet." We say it with a sheepish look of apology or a shrug of the shoulders. Though we may or may not say it aloud and may not even realize we are thinking it, we take those thoughts even further and think, "Not long after I finish my diet, I will join you in complete indulgence and forget my health and wellbeing."

We don't say it, but we feel like a social outcast on a diet. We secretly are counting the days until we can return to being part of the social norm. Thinking like this will not help you make lifetime choices. With thinking like this, you have already decided you are making these dietary choices on a limited basis and will return to what you believe to be normal in due time. This kind of thinking is self-defeating. You need to change this way of thinking. One way is to take steps to avoid feeling like a social outcast. Call a friend and share your new menu. Share what you are doing and invite your friend to a lunch or dinner that you make from your acceptable food list.

Write a reflection of this experience with your friend.

Exercise 14.2

Write your gratitude entry, the ten things that went well today, and your daily present-tense, positive affirmations.

I am grateful for…

_____

_____

_____

_____

_____

_____

10 Things I Did Well Today

1. _____
2. _____
3. _____
4. _____
5. _____
6. _____
7. _____
8. _____
9. _____
10. _____

Daily Positive Affirmations:

1. _____
   _____
2. _____
   _____
3. _____
   _____

Exercise 14.3

Keep your food diary.

Breakfast:_____

Snack: _____

Lunch: _____

Dinner: _____

Snack: _____

Drinks:_____

Water Intake: _____

Action Steps: DAY 15

Exercise 15.1

Make a plan to treat yourself to a non-food reward. You have been making tremendous strides in your goals. It is time to reward yourself. The goal here is to do something just for you that feels empowering, feels rewarding, and is not food. Examples are: going to a movie you really want to see, buying that new bestseller you can put in your sacred space or emergency kit, or it can be even simpler like a new pair of earrings or a new shade of lipstick for the new and evolving you.

Write a reflection on this experience in two parts, the first part on planning the reward and the second on the completion of the experience.

_____

_____

_____

_____

_____

_____

_____

_____

_____

_____

_____

_____

_____

_____

_____

_____

Exercise 15.2

Write your gratitude entry, the ten things that went well today, and your daily present-tense, positive affirmations.

I am grateful for...

_____

_____

_____

_____

_____

_____

10 Things I Did Well Today

1. _____
2. _____
3. _____
4. _____
5. _____
6. _____

7. 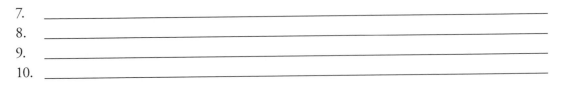_____

8. _____

9. _____

10. _____

Daily Positive Affirmations:

1. _____
   _____

2. _____
   _____

3. _____
   _____

Exercise 15.3

Keep your food diary.

Breakfast: _____

Snack: _____

Lunch: _____

Dinner: _____

Snack: _____

Drinks:_____

Water Intake: _____

Action Steps: DAY 16

Exercise 16.1

Change your computer wallpaper. This is a fabulous visualization exercise. Create a folder in your computer in your pictures folder. Name this folder "Visualization." In it, put at least a dozen images of photos that represent the best of your current life. Add at least a dozen images of photos that you get from the internet that represent future goals, wishes and dreams. You can even include some of the clothing of the size you are working toward. You can choose photos of places you want to visit, of healthy meals that look and taste delicious, or even of the car you hope to have. Anything. The possibilities are endless.

Look in this folder often for encouragement or make a slide show on your computer. If you don't know how to do this, search how to set a slide show as your wallpaper in your computer's Help function. Set the timer to rotate the picture every 10-30 seconds, whatever you choose. Now when you play your slide show, your computer will help penetrate your mind with these healthy images, keeping you motivated and focused on the positives instead of the negatives.

Exercise 16.2

Write your gratitude entry, the ten things that went well today, and your daily present-tense, positive affirmations.

I am grateful for…

_____

_____

_____

_____

_____

_____

10 Things I Did Well Today

1. _____
2. _____
3. _____
4. _____
5. _____
6. _____
7. _____
8. _____
9. _____
10. _____

Daily Positive Affirmations:

1. _____

_____

2. _____

_____

3. _____
   _____

Exercise 16.3

Keep your food diary.

Breakfast: _____
Snack: _____
Lunch: _____
Dinner: _____
Snack: _____
Drinks:_____
Water Intake: _____

Action Steps: DAY 17

Exercise 17.1

Change the music in your car. This may seem like a totally irrelevant action step, but it can make a difference in how you handle stress which will then influence your health. Think about it. The car is actually a place where we typically have way too much going on. All at the same time, kids or other passengers are talking; music is playing; a DVD player or gaming device is making background noise; either you or someone else may be talking on the phone, or you may have a lot on your mind—not to mention that if you are driving, you also need to deal with the actual mental and physical stress of driving on the streets and paying attention to other drivers. How many times do we add eating to that potentially dangerous mix?

Driving can be an activity where we are majorly over stimulated, and we fail to breathe well and focus on the task at hand. If you learn how to minimize the overstimulation, you see how there are different strategies for dealing with stress. Maybe then you can see the potential for avoiding eating in stressful scenarios. The first step to do this is to turn the music in your car to something relaxing (with little to no talk or advertisements) or turn it off altogether. You will be amazed at how your stress levels while driving change.

Set a reminder on your phone to come back to Exercise 17.1 after you have had a few chances to drive with the changes you make. When you return, write a reflection on this experience.

Exercise 17.2

Write your gratitude entry, the ten things that went well today, and your daily present-tense, positive affirmations.

I am grateful for…

_____
_____
_____
_____

10 Things I Did Well Today

1. _____
2. _____
3. _____
4. _____
5. _____
6. _____
7. _____
8. _____
9. _____
10. _____

Daily Positive Affirmations:

1. _____
   _____
2. _____
   _____
3. _____
   _____

Exercise 17.3

Keep your food diary.

Breakfast: _____
Snack: _____
Lunch: _____
Dinner: _____
Snack: _____
Drinks:_____
Water Intake: _____

Action Steps: DAY 18

Exercise 18.1

Go to bed early. Your health and weight issues will not get better without enough good rest. Good rest is seven to eight hours of uninterrupted sleep. When you are overly tired and do not sleep, there is a greater tendency to want to eat. Our bodies need the rest to help our bodies detoxify and rejuvenate. Tonight, or tomorrow night if you are reading this too late tonight, make the commitment to be in bed by 10:00 or 10:30 pm or whatever time will allow you to sleep for seven to eight hours before your next day begins. Challenge yourself to keep this bedtime for two weeks straight and see how good being rested can feel.

Set a reminder to return to Exercise 18.1 to write a reflection upon how refreshed and less stressed you are when getting enough sleep.

Exercise 18.2

Write your gratitude entry, ten things that went well today and your daily present-tense, positive affirmations.

I am grateful for…

_____

_____

_____

_____

_____

_____

_____

10 Things I Did Well Today

1. _____
2. _____
3. _____
4. _____
5. _____
6. _____
7. _____
8. _____
9. _____
10. _____

Daily Positive Affirmations:

1. _____
   _____
2. _____
   _____
3. _____
   _____

Exercise 18.3

Keep your food diary.

Breakfast: _____
Snack: _____
Lunch: _____
Dinner: _____
Snack: _____
Drinks:_____
Water Intake: _____
Bedtime: _____

Action Steps: DAY 19

Exercise 19.1

You can say no. This exercise is not about saying no to food, it is about reflecting on times when failing to say no in other situations costs your health. Saying no is one of the most challenging things to do for anyone who wants to put everyone else's needs ahead of her own. If you overeat because you overextend yourself, then now is a good time to think about how this may be affecting your health.

Write about a time when you did not say no, but maybe you should have. How may have it affected your health?

_____
_____
_____
_____
_____
_____
_____
_____
_____
_____
_____
_____
_____
_____
_____
_____
_____
_____

Exercise 19.2

Write your gratitude entry, ten things that went well today and your daily present-tense, positive affirmations.

I am grateful for…

_____
_____
_____
_____
_____
_____

10 Things I Did Well Today

1. _____
2. _____
3. _____
4. _____
5. _____

6. _____

7. _____

8. _____

9. _____

10. _____

Daily Positive Affirmations:

1. _____
   _____

2. _____
   _____

3. _____
   _____

Exercise 19.3

Keep your food diary.

Breakfast: _____

Snack: _____

Lunch: _____

Dinner: _____

Snack: _____

Drinks:_____

Water Intake: _____

Bedtime:_____

Action Steps: DAY 20

Exercise 20.1

Write a letter to the new you. Praise and encourage her for her efforts and her progress. You can write this letter on your computer, or you can write it here or in your notebook where you can reflect upon it at a later time.

Dear New Me,

_____

_____

_____

_____

_____

_____

_____

Exercise 20.2

Write your gratitude entry, ten things that went well today and your daily present-tense, positive affirmations.

I am grateful for…

_____

_____

_____

_____

_____

_____

10 Things I Did Well Today

1. _____
2. _____
3. _____
4. _____
5. _____
6. _____
7. _____
8. _____
9. _____
10. _____

Daily Positive Affirmations:

1. _____

_____

2. _____
   _____

3. _____
   _____

Exercise 20.3

Keep your food diary.

Breakfast: _____
Snack: _____
Lunch: _____
Dinner: _____
Snack: _____
Drinks:_____
Water Intake: _____
Bedtime: _____

Actions Steps: DAY 21

Exercise 21.1

Give yourself a hug. You are amazing and deserve to take small moments *daily* to recognize your work and support yourself with love. Write a reflection of this experience and what it means to you to be recognizing your efforts in small ways.

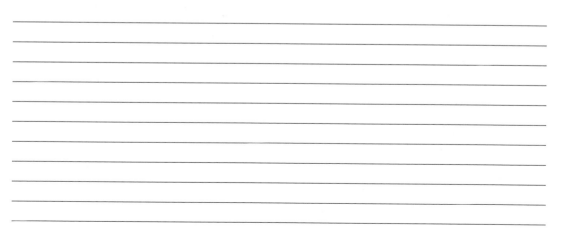

Exercise 21.2

Write your gratitude entry, ten things that went well today and your daily present-tense, positive affirmations.

I am grateful for…

10 Things I Did Well Today

1. _____
2. _____
3. _____
4. _____

5. _____
6. _____
7. _____
8. _____
9. _____
10. _____

Daily Positive Affirmations:

1. _____
_____

2. _____
_____

3. _____
_____

Exercise 21.3

Keep your food diary.

Breakfast: _____
Snack: _____
Lunch: _____
Dinner: _____
Snack: _____
Drinks:_____
Water Intake: _____
Bedtime: _____

CONCLUSION

Congratulations! You are on well on your way to your best self! They say it takes twenty-one days to make or break a habit. The hope is that, with these twenty-one days of thought-filled exercises and experiences, you have made a strong commitment to your health and well-being. You have done the mental and emotional work to help jumpstart your success.

Continue to use your Linked food resources to create each week's menu plan and grocery list, write your gratitude and food diary entries daily, and complete any exercises that you have not yet finished. Be patient with yourself and love yourself well. Take everything one day at a time. Return to or repeat any other exercise that was meaningful and purposeful to your health and well-being as you need during your journey. Don't worry if you find yourself repeating exercises multiple times before reaching your goals. Each time you return to an exercise, or your Linked Diet Food List or any other recommendations made in this book, you are learning to build a permanently new you with a full and vibrant life.

If you find yourself really struggling and need professional help, you can find out more about my services and schedule a phone or in person appointment on my website at www.laurakopec.com.

Cheers to the new you and your best self!

Linked TYPE A Food List and Supplements

60% of food	*40% of food*	*NOT AT ALL*
Fruit: ALL (except banana, grapes, oranges and tomatoes) **Vegetables:** ALL (except peas) **Nuts:** Almonds **Grains/Starches:** Fingerling potatoes Acorn or Butternut Squash Quinoa Tapioca **Small amounts of:** Flax and Flax oil Coconut and Coconut Oil Extra-virgin Olive Oil	**Dairy:** Cage-free/organic eggs (pasture-fed is ideal) **Seafood:** Shrimp, Mussels, Wild Salmon and Other Fish (except Tuna) **Meats:** Organic chicken Turkey and Lamb **Nuts:** Pistachios, Walnuts Raw Cashews (not roasted in peanut oil) **Other:** Brown or Basmati Rice Black, Navy and Lima beans Raw honey	**Fruit/Vegetables:** Produce imported from non-European countries **Starches:** Gluten (no wheat or white flour foods) Enriched or white rice **Dairy:** Cow dairy (all except organic butter) **Meats:** Red meat (Beef or Buffalo) Pork (ham, bacon, pork chops, pork loin, etc.) Lobster Crab Tuna **Oils:** Corn and corn oil Canola oil Soybean oil Hydrogenated and partially hydrogenated oils **Sugars and Sweeteners:** White and brown sugar Aspartame, NutraSweet, Equal, Sweet n Low and Splenda Agave Nectar High fructose corn syrup Dextrose and Maltodextrin **Other:** Dough conditioners MSG Autolyzed yeast protein Autolyzed soy protein Beer

One time per week

AT MOST once every 4 days

Fruit/Vegetables: Bananas, Grapes, Oranges and Raisins, Peas Tomatoes **Starches:** White, red, yellow or sweet potatoes **Meats:** Chicken (cage free or range free, avoid regular chicken altogether)	**Dairy:** Goat products (goat feta, goat yogurt, goat milk) Organic butter (from cow's milk) **Other:** Pinto and Kidney Organic Soy beans Peanuts Agave Nectar

Guidelines to Increase Your Body's Response:

- Begin your morning with adequate fiber such as oats, flax seed or flax meal and fruit.
- Consume your largest meal at lunch and a full-sized salad containing light protein such as egg or seafood for dinner. If you prepare a large dinner for your family that fits your food recommendations, save your portion and eat it for lunch the next day.
- Do not eat more than two servings of animal protein a day.

Supplemental Considerations for Linked Type A

Supplements are key components of your Linked Diet. Foundational supplements, like multivitamins and minerals, are essential to maintain healthy nutritional levels and are intended for life-long use. Clean and repair supplements are NOT intended to be life-long supplements. Instead, they work to more quickly restore nutritional deficiencies that, without supplementation, may slowly and eventually disappear as proper foods are eaten consistently (resulting in the digestive changes needed to restore balance to the body.)

The best way to ensure you are getting the correct supplements that coincide with your Linked Type and your biochemical individuality is to consult with a nutritionist or other healthcare professional that specializes in this area. And remember, it is always a good idea to have your doctor's approval before making any dietary changes or taking any supplements to avoid any complications or unknown contraindications with medications. Please note supplement recommendations are not approved for women who are pregnant or nursing, adults who are taking prescription medications, or minors under the age of 18.

Consider the following supplements to enhance your Linked Type A food protocol:

- *A good multivitamin and mineral supplement.*
  A basic multivitamin may not have minerals. Read the label to make sure your multivitamin also contains these important minerals: calcium, magnesium, potassium, phosphorus, iodine, zinc, and selenium. Minerals are as equally important to a well-rounded supplement as vitamins.
- *Extra magnesium paired with a multivitamin that has calcium.*
  This may be an important piece to help move things along while restoring your digestive health. Extra magnesium in addition to a multivitamin and mineral supplement that already contains calcium and magnesium can help you have daily bowel movements as well as improve bowel function and ease. If daily bowel movements are not happening, then weight loss can be stunted. Try an additional 100–200mg of magnesium glycinate or magnesium citrate every night before bed in addition to your multivitamin. The extra

magnesium may or may not be needed after you lose the weight to keep your bowel movements regular. Be sure to eat plenty of good fruits and vegetables while taking the magnesium to get good fiber.

- *Extra Vitamin C in a range of 500-2000mg.*

  If you feel as if you still need an extra boost to get daily bowel movements, or need to give yourself some additional immune support, then extra Vitamin C may be appropriate. The extra Vitamin C should not give you diarrhea. If it does, the dose is likely too high. Start with 500mg (typically one pill, capsule or tablet) and increase the dosage each day until you have soft and loose stools without diarrhea. Linked Type A often has constipation issues, and the combination of magnesium and Vitamin C is often a good fit.

- *A probiotic with at least eight strains of bacteria that cumulatively account for over one billion organisms.*

  A high-potency probiotic is absolutely essential and foundational for everyone from infants to seniors and should be taken permanently. A probiotic should have at least eight different strains of bacteria, and total of over one billion organisms. Probiotics contain live, helpful bacteria and many require refrigeration. Only buy probiotics from companies or health care professionals that guarantee the potency.

- *A comprehensive digestive enzyme.*

  The body may need help digesting carbohydrates, protein and fat as well as help balancing metabolism during weight loss. Digestive enzymes should be taken temporarily while you are losing the weight if you are under the age of 40; otherwise, a dependency could occur. Following your food plan well will help the body once again produce the enzymes adequately on its own. After the age of 40, a digestive enzyme may be necessary for continued optimal health as normal enzyme function depletes as we age. If you are Linked Type A, your digestive enzyme supplement should contain enzymes to assist with proteins such as protease, pepsin and betaine hcl; enzymes to help with fats such as lipase; and enzymes to help with carbohydrates such as amylase.

- *Super foods or super supplements.*

  Consider taking aloe vera juice, which will act as a great restorer to the digestive tract. This juice helps soothe the stomach lining and intestinal membranes and may have a truly positive affect on your weight. Aloe vera juice can be taken as the label recommends.

Linked TYPE A Sample Meal Plan

	BREAKFAST (Fiber)	LUNCH (Main meal)	SNACK (Protein and fruit)	DINNER (Light meal)
SUN	½ c gluten-free oatmeal with 1 TB flax meal and ¼ c blueberries 1 c green tea with 2 TB unsweetened almond milk	4 oz turkey breast, baked or sautéed in coconut oil ½ c steamed broccoli ½ c cooked yellow lentils with fresh garlic and ginger	1 raw apple ½ c walnuts	Mixed-greens salad: shredded carrot ¼ c sliced almonds Serve with 2 oz wild salmon, baked or poached. Drizzle extra-virgin olive oil and squeeze ¼ lemon
MON	½ c gluten free oatmeal with 1 TB flax meal and ¼ c blackberries 1 c Earl Grey tea with 2 TB unsweetened almond milk	1 Lamb chop, pan-fried in coconut oil 1 c Navy beans ½ c wilted spinach tossed in extra-virgin olive oil and sprinkled with sea salt	1 hard-boiled egg 1 raw apple ¼ c pistachios	Smoothie in blender: ½ c unsweetened almond milk 2 TB almond butter 2 TB unsweetened cocoa powder ¼ c raw cashews
TUES	1 baked apple stuffed with chopped pecans, sprinkled with cinnamon 1 c chamomile tea	1 Tilapia sautéed in coconut oil 1 cucumber, sliced 1 avocado, sliced ½ c broccoli, steamed	Goat cheese 1 raw pear or nectarine	1 large baked sweet potato drizzled with extra-virgin olive oil and sprinkled with sea salt
WED	1 c cooked Arrowhead Rice and Shine® ½ c blueberries 1 c green tea with 1 tsp raw honey	1 c basmati or brown rice ½ c black beans 1 avocado 1 TB chopped tomato	2 stalks of celery washed and cut into pieces with almond butter	2-egg omelet with 1 sliced red bell pepper
THUR	½ c gluten free oatmeal with 1 TB flax meal, 1 TB unsweetened, apple sauce, and ½ tsp cinnamon	4 large shrimp sauteed in extra-virgin olive oil served with 1-2 c stir fry of onion, zucchini and red bell pepper	1 raw apple with almond butter	Smoothie: ½ c unsweetened almond milk ½ c frozen or fresh strawberries, 2 TB almond butter
FRI	½ c gluten free oatmeal with 1 TB flax meal, ½ c strawberries 1 c black tea with 2 TB almond milk	1 turkey burger wrapped in lettuce with 1 avocado 1 c sweet potato fries, baked	2 oz smoked or poached salmon and 4 sliced radishes	2 hard-boiled eggs 1 apple
SAT	Fruit bowl: 1 apple ½ c blueberries ½ c strawberries ½ c diced pineapple 1 c chamomile tea	Food 4 Life® brown rice tortilla with goat cheese cooked as a quesadilla 1 c spinach with chopped mushrooms and red onion	Hard-boiled egg ½ c pistachios	1 c blackberries with ¼ c coconut cream poured over

Linked Type A Breakfast Recipes

Baked Apple Delight

Ingredients:
4 large apples peeled, cored and sliced
½ cup raw honey, divided
½ cup almond meal/flour
½ cup oats
¼ cup ground flax
½ cup extra-virgin olive oil

Preheat oven to 350°F. Peel, core and slice apples and arrange on bottom of 9x13x2-inch, glass casserole dish. Drizzle ¼ cup of honey over apples. Decrease oven temperature to 300°F to avoid overheating extra-virgin olive oil. Bake apples for approximately 20 minutes.

Take out of oven. Keep oven temperature at 300°F.

In a separate bowl, mix almond meal, oats, flax and olive oil until crumbly. Sprinkle mixture on top of apples. Drizzle remaining ¼ cup of honey over crumbs. Bake apple crisp for 10-15 minutes or until topping is browned to your satisfaction.

Serve warm or at room temperature. Apple crisp is traditionally thought of as a dessert, but with all healthy ingredients you can prepare this the night before and have breakfast ready to go first thing in the morning.

Breakfast Muffins

Ingredients:
1 cups gluten-free flour
2 teaspoons baking powder
½ teaspoon flax seed meal
½ teaspoon cinnamon
½ teaspoon sea salt
¼ teaspoon baking soda
½ cup olive oil (or goat butter on your once a week)
½ cup raw honey
3 large cage-free eggs

1 cup unsweetened apple sauce
½ cup almond pieces
½ cup dried, shredded coconut (optional)

Preheat oven to 350°F. Grease a 12-cup muffin pan with coconut oil (if using papers, grease papers.) In a large mixing bowl, add gluten-free flour, baking powder, flax seed meal, cinnamon, sea salt and baking soda. Stir together and set aside. In a blender, add apple sauce, oil and honey. Blend. Add eggs and blend again. Add blended mixture to dry ingredients. Mix well. Stir in nuts and coconut. Spoon batter into greased muffin pan.

Reduce heat in oven to 325°F. Bake for 20-25 minutes. Remove from oven and let cool 5 minutes before removing from pan.

Enjoy warm or refrigerate or freeze for later in airtight container.

Hearty Granola

Ingredients:
2 cups rolled oats
1 cup uncooked quinoa
1 cup slivered or sliced almonds
1 cup raw pumpkin seeds
½ cup raw sunflower seeds
¼ cup flax seed or golden flax seed
1 cup raw, unprocessed honey
1 cup filtered water
1 cup extra-virgin olive oil

Preheat oven to 350°F. In a very large mixing bowl or large stock pot, add all dry ingredients. Set aside. In a medium saucepan, combine honey, water and oil. Simmer until liquid ingredients are well combined. Slowly pour liquids into stock pot, stirring constantly to keep liquid from over saturating any one part of dry ingredients.
Spread mixture onto a greased baking sheet. Reduce heat and bake at 325°F for approximately 10-15 minutes or until granola starts to brown. Take out of oven and let cool.

After it is completely cooled, granola can be stored in a large container. Serve with your favorite milk (goat or almond) or with a plain goat yogurt. If desired, add fresh fruit when serving to increase nutritional content.

Rustic Porridge

Make 4-6 servings.

Ingredients:
2 cups unsweetened almond milk
¼ teaspoon sea salt
1 cup steel cut oats
½ cup uncooked quinoa
½ cup slivered almonds
½ cup blackberries
½ cup blueberries
¼ teaspoon cinnamon

In a medium saucepan, bring almond milk and salt to a low boil. Add oats and quinoa. Slow cook for 30-45 minutes or until milk is absorbed and porridge is the desired consistency.

Spoon out into bowls. Divide almonds, blackberries and blueberries over the top. Sprinkle with cinnamon.

HINT: For a shorter cook time, replace steel cut oats with Scottish oats.

Breakfast Fruit and Nut Bars

Ingredients:
1 cup dates or figs
1 cup dried cherries
¼ cup raw cashews

Put all ingredients into a large food processor and mix until mixture begins to clump or ball up. Remove and form into bars or balls.

Place in snack-size re-sealable bags or roll up in wax paper. Store in refrigerator.

Tropical Smoothie

Ingredients:
½ cup unsweetened almond milk
1 banana
½ cup pineapple (fresh or frozen)
½ cup mango (fresh or frozen)
2 tablespoon shredded, unsweetened coconut

Place ingredients in blender. Blend until smooth.

Serve immediately.

HINT: Can add ½ cup ice before blending for a different consistency.

Linked Type A Lunch Recipes

Black Beans and Quinoa

Ingredients
1 cup dried quinoa
1 small can black beans
¼ red onion, diced
1 avocado, cut into chunks
2 tablespoon extra-virgin olive oil
1 tablespoon Bragg apple cider vinegar
Romaine lettuce leaves

In a medium saucepan, add 2 cups of filtered water and quinoa. Bring to a boil. Boil for 10 minutes. Cover and remove from heat to let water absorb.

Drain and rinse black beans in small strainer. Dice the red onion into very small pieces and set aside. In a large mixing bowl, mix black beans, red onion, and avocado. Add olive oil and vinegar.

When quinoa is cooked, rinse in a tight weave strainer under cold water for a minute or so. Pour quinoa into bowl with beans and other ingredients. Toss lightly to mix but not crush the avocado. Serve immediately on a leaf of Romaine lettuce. Works well with leftover quinoa. If preparing in advance, wait to cut and add avocado until just before serving to keep avocado pieces from turning grey or brown.

Egg Salad Surprise

Ingredients
1 cup cooked brown rice
2 hard boiled eggs
¼ cup roasted or raw sunflower seeds
2 tablespoons dried parsley
1 cucumber
1 radish
2 tablespoons extra-virgin olive oil
1 tablespoons Bragg apple cider vinegar
Butter lettuce (optional)

In a large mixing bowl, add rice, egg, sunflower seeds, parsley, olive oil and vinegar. Toss. Peel cucumber. Slice long and scoop out seeds with spoon and discard. Dice cucumber into bite size pieces and add to the egg salad. Dice radish and add to the mixture.

Serve immediately or refrigerate for later. Can be served plain on a plate or over butter lettuce.

Fish Tacos

Ingredients
2 tilapia filets
1 mango, sliced
¼ cup raw cabbage, shredded
1 avocado, sliced
2 Food 4 Life® brown rice tortillas
1 tablespoons coconut oil

Warm coconut oil in large skillet. Add tilapia filets. Sea salt and pepper generously. Brown on both sides. When cooked, place on a dish and cover.

In the same skillet, warm each side of each tortilla to soften. Place one tortilla each on a large dinner plate. Place half of the cabbage on one side of each tortilla. Place avocado and mango evenly on top of cabbage. Break up one tilapia filet and top one tortilla. Break up remaining filet and top remaining tortilla. Fold tortillas in half. Cut each in half to make 4 tacos.

Pineapple Fried Rice

Ingredients
1 cup cooked rice (or quinoa)
1 cup carrots, grated
¼ red onion, diced small
1 cup peas, frozen or fresh
2 eggs
½ cup diced pineapple
1 tablespoon coconut oil
Sea salt
Pepper

In a large skillet, add coconut oil, rice, carrots, onion, peas. Beat eggs in small bowl before adding to the rice and veggies. Sea salt and pepper to taste. Stir often, but allow to slightly brown on one side. At the last few minutes, add the pineapple. If using canned pineapple in own juices, drain before adding. Serve hot.

Quick Tilapia and Greens

Ingredients:
Tilapia filet (1 per person) (can use Rainbow trout)
1 tablespoon coconut oil
Sea salt
Black Pepper
Red bell pepper
1 cup chopped kale or spinach
Sliced almonds
Extra-virgin olive oil

In a large skillet melt the coconut oil. Lay tilapia on melted oil. Sprinkle generously with sea salt and pepper. Brown on both sides. Set aside and keep warm.

While cooking the fish, slice a red bell pepper very thin. Remove seeds and stem. After removing fish, add red pepper to hot skillet. Sautee and add chopped greens. Remove from pan. Drizzle with olive oil, and sprinkle with almonds. Add fish over the top.

Serve immediately.

Salmon Patties

Ingredients:
1 can of pink salmon
2 slices of EnerG® tapioca bread
¼ cup unsweetened almond milk
1 cage free egg
1 teaspoon Annie's Naturals® yellow mustard
Sea salt
Black pepper
1 tablespoon coconut oil
Sliced jicama
Sliced strawberries
Spinach

Open the can of salmon. Remove the large bones from the salmon and leave the little bones. Set aside.

In a large bowl, break bread into pieces or crumbs. Add milk. Mix well. Add salmon, egg, mustard, sea salt and pepper. Mix ingredients with your hands until completely blended. Shape into patties.

In a large skillet, melt coconut oil and place the salmon patties in the skillet. When browned on one side, flip and brown on the other side.

Serve with spinach, strawberries and jicama.

Stuffed Avocado with Smoked Salmon

2 ounces smoked salmon (or smoked trout)
1 celery stalk, diced
2 tablespoons red onion, diced

1 tablespoon extra-virgin olive oil
1 avocado
1 carrot, sliced
1 apple, sliced
Sea salt
Black pepper

In a medium mixing bowl, break up the salmon into bite size pieces. Add celery, onion, and olive oil. Salt and pepper to taste. Slice avocado in half lengthwise and remove pit. Add a spoonful of salmon salad to the center of each avocado half.

Serve with carrot and apple on the side. Use 1 avocado per person. Salmon salad can be made in advance for future use.

Linked Type A Dinner Recipes

Shrimp Lettuce Wraps

Makes 4 wraps

Ingredients:
½ pound shrimp, peeled and deveined
2 tablespoons coconut oil
1 carrot, julienned
1 green zucchini, julienned
1 yellow crookneck squash, julienned
Red leaf lettuce
Sea salt
Black pepper

In a medium skillet, sauté shrimp in coconut oil. Add sea salt and pepper to taste. While shrimp is cooking, lay zucchini and crook-neck squash evenly on a paper towel. Sprinkle with salt. Leave for 5-10 minutes. (This process will pull moisture out of the veggies and keep them crisp.) Rinse and pat dry. Place in bowl. Add carrots. Set aside.

Pull lettuce off the stem being careful not to break. Wash and pat dry. Lay lettuce sheet on a plate. Add spoonful of cooked shrimp and spoonful of veggies. Tuck the ends of the lettuce in and roll the lettuce around to create a wrap.

Serve immediately. Can serve with sliced apples or pears or alone.

Chef's Salad

Ingredients:
1 head romaine lettuce
1 large carrot, shredded
2 eggs, hardboiled
¼ cup almonds, sliced
1 Gala apple, cored and sliced
1 tablespoons extra-virgin olive oil
½ lemon

Dice romaine lettuce and place on large platter. Shred carrot and sprinkle evenly over the lettuce. Peel and slice hardboiled egg and lay over the lettuce. Sprinkle almond over the top. Arrange apple slices over the mixture. Drizzle with olive oil, and squeeze lemon over the top.

Deviled Eggs with Veggies

Ingredients:
2 cage free eggs, hard-boiled
3 tablespoons Annie's Naturals® yellow mustard
4 tablespoons extra-virgin olive oil
1 teaspoon dried parsley
¼ teaspoon sea salt
¼ teaspoon black pepper
¼ teaspoon paprika
1 carrot, sliced
1 cucumber, sliced
Butter or Red Lettuce

Best to hard-boil eggs a day ahead: In a medium stockpot, cover raw eggs with water. Bring to a boil. Boil for 10 minutes. Turn off heat and remove pot from burner. Let sit until water has cooled down. Take eggs out of water and refrigerate, if boiled early.

Peel hardboiled eggs. Slice egg whites lengthwise around yolks to cleanly open each white into 2 halves. Lay whites on flat plate or platter. Place yolks in medium mixing bowl. Add mustard, olive oil, parsley, sea salt and pepper. Mix until creamy.

Place 1 heaping teaspoon of the creamy yolk mixture into each egg white half. Sprinkle each with a pinch of paprika. Refrigerate.

Best served chilled with side salad of lettuce, carrot, cucumber drizzled with olive oil and sprinkled with sea salt.

Veggie Stir Fry

Ingredients:
2 cups water, filtered
1 cup quinoa, uncooked
2 carrots, sliced
1 green bell pepper, diced
½ red onion, cut in large chunks
1 tablespoons coconut oil
2 tablespoons almonds, slivered
1 Gala apple, sliced with skin
Sea salt
Black pepper

In a medium sauce pan, bring water to a boil. Add quinoa and return to a boil. Reduce heat for 5 minutes. Remove from heat and cover. Let sit until water is absorbed.

In a large skillet, warm coconut oil. Add carrots, green bell pepper and red onion. Sauté until desired texture is reached. Add sea salt and black pepper to taste. Sprinkle with almonds.

Serve over cooked quinoa with apple slices laid on top.

Shrimp Scampi Salad with Broccoli Side

Ingredients:
2 tablespoons coconut oil
3 cloves fresh garlic, minced
1 pound Gulf shrimp, peeled and deveined

1 head of broccoli, diced very small
1 bunch of green onions, diced
1 head of butter lettuce, sliced
1 ripe avocado, sliced
Sea salt
Pepper

Pour coconut oil in large skillet. Add garlic. Cook for 1 minute. Add shrimp and sauté until shrimp is fully cooked, turning often. Remove from skillet, cover and set aside. Add onion and broccoli to skillet. Toss while cooking for 1 minute or until broccoli is bright green and tender. Do not overcook. Salt and pepper to taste.

Serve shrimp over lettuce and avocado with broccoli on the side.

Quinoa Salad

Ingredients:
1 cup quinoa
1 cucumber
1 red bell pepper
2 tablespoon goat feta cheese, divided
¼ c pitted Kalamata black olives
Extra-virgin olive oil
1 lemon
Romaine lettuce

In a medium saucepan, add water and quinoa. Bring to a boil. Boil for 10 minutes. Cover and remove from heat. Let stand until water is absorbed.

Meanwhile, peel and cut cucumber lengthwise. Scoop seeds out with spoon, discard. Chop cucumber. Cut open red bell pepper. Remove and discard seeds. Dice bell pepper. Crumble or dice a small portion of feta cheese just as needed.

Run quinoa under cold water in tight strainer to cool quinoa. In a large mixing bowl, add cooled quinoa, cucumber, red bell pepper, and remaining feta cheese. Drain olives, if needed, and add desired amount to salad. Drizzle with olive oil, and squeeze lemon over top. Toss.

Serve over romaine lettuce leaf.

Linked TYPE B Food List and Supplements

80% of food	*20%* of food	*NOT AT ALL*
Fruit: ALL (except bananas and grapes)	*Dairy:* Cage-free/organic eggs (pasture-fed is ideal)	*Fruit/Vegetables:* Produce imported from non-European countries
Vegetables: ALL (except peas) Dark leafy greens (Spinach, arugula, kale, chard, turnip greens, etc.)	*Seafood:* Shrimp Mussels Wild Salmon and Fish	*Starches:* Enriched or white rice Gluten (no wheat or white flour foods)
Nuts: Almonds Raw cashews	*Meats:* Organic chicken Turkey Lamb	*Dairy:* Cow dairy (all except organic butter)
Grains/Starches: Oats Fingerling potatoes Acorn or Butternut Squash Tapioca	*Nuts:* Pistachios and Walnuts *Other:* Brown or Basmati Rice Black, Navy and Lima beans Lentils Raw honey	*Meats:* Red meat (Beef or Buffalo) Pork (ham, bacon, pork chops, pork loin, etc.) Lobster Crab Tuna
Other: Flax and Flax Oil Extra-virgin Olive Oil		*Other:* Peanuts Corn (and corn oil) Canola oil Soybean oil Hydrogenated and partially hydrogenated oils White and brown sugar, Aspartame, NutraSweet, Equal, Sweet n Low, Splenda High fructose corn syrup, Dextrose, Maltodextrin Agave Nectar Dough conditioners MSG Autolyzed yeast protein Autolyzed soy protein

One time per week
AT MOST once every 4 days

Fruit/Vegetables: Bananas, Grapes Oranges, Raisins Peas and Tomatoes	*Dairy*: Goat products (goat feta, goat yogurt, goat milk) Organic butter (from cow's milk)	
Starches: Sweet potatoes White, red, yellow or sweet potatoes	*Other*: Pinto and Kidney beans Organic Soy beans Coconut and coconut oil	
Meats: Chicken (cage free/range free or organic)		

Guidelines to Increase Your Body's Response:

- Begin each day, 20 minutes before having breakfast, with this morning tonic: 8 ounces of water with 2 ounces of aloe vera juice and liquid chlorophyll (follow label recommendations for a single serving on the brand you purchase), a pinch of pink Himalayan sea salt, and one-half of a lemon-freshly squeezed.
- Consume your larger meal at lunch. If you prepare a large dinner for your family that also meets your food list recommendations, take your portion as leftovers and eat for lunch.
- Consume a full size salad for dinner containing light protein such as egg or seafood.
- Do not eat more than 1–2 servings of animal protein a day. Consume complete proteins (protein with good carbohydrate) of beans and rice (or goat cheese within your weekly limit) for protein.
- Cook with herbs and spices such as cinnamon, garlic and pink Himalayan sea salt
- Drink an 8 ounce glass of water with 1 teaspoon of Bragg Apple Cider Vinegar between 3:00 pm and 5:00 pm each day.

Supplement Considerations for Linked Type B

Supplements are key components of your Linked Diet. Foundational supplements, like multivitamins and minerals, are essential to maintain healthy nutritional levels and are intended for life-long use. Clean and repair supplements are NOT intended to be life-long supplements. Instead, they work to more quickly restore nutritional deficiencies that, without supplementation, may slowly and eventually disappear as proper foods are eaten consistently (resulting in the digestive changes needed to restore balance to the body.)

The best way to ensure you are getting the correct supplements that coincide with your Linked Type and your biochemical individuality is to consult with a nutritionist or other healthcare professional that specializes in this area. And remember, it is always a good idea to have your doctor's approval before making any dietary changes or taking any supplements to avoid any complications or unknown contraindications with medications. Please note supplement recommendations are not approved for women who are pregnant or nursing, adults who are taking prescription medications, or minors under the age of 18.

Consider the following supplements to enhance your Linked Type B food protocol:

- *A good multivitamin and mineral supplement.*
  A general vitamin may not have minerals, so read the label to make sure your multivitamin also contains these important minerals: calcium, magnesium, potassium, phosphorus, zinc and selenium. Minerals are as equally important to a well-rounded supplement.

- *A probiotic with at least eight strains of bacteria that cumulatively account for over one billion organisms.*

  A high-potency probiotic is absolutely essential and foundational for everyone from infants to seniors and should be taken permanently. A probiotic should have at least eight different strains of bacteria, and total of over one billion organisms. Probiotics contain live, helpful bacteria and many require refrigeration. Only buy probiotics from companies or health care professionals that guarantee the potency.

- *Extra magnesium.*

  This may be an important piece to help move things along while restoring your digestive health. Extra magnesium in addition to a multivitamin and mineral supplement that already contains calcium and magnesium can help you have daily bowel movements as well as improve bowel function and ease. If daily bowel movements are not happening, then weight loss can be stunted. Try an additional 100–200mg of magnesium glycinate or magnesium citrate every night before bed in addition to your multivitamin. The extra magnesium may or may not be needed after you lose the weight to keep your bowel movements regular. Be sure to eat plenty of good fruits and vegetables while taking the magnesium to get good fiber.

- *Glutathione, a major antioxidant.*

  When the body is weighted down with a high toxic load, as may be the case in the Linked Type B individual, there may not be enough glutathione for the body to be functioning optimally. Glutathione is a major antioxidant that helps the body clear toxins such as heavy metals, dietary toxins, and pollutants. Glutathione also helps restore cells, recover from oxidative stress and fight infection. While glutathione is found in foods such as walnuts and apples, a supplement may improve your body's ability to detoxify and recover from physical stressors. A supplement containing approximately 100–150 mg of glutathione per day may be appropriate if you are Linked Type B, and you are not taking any prescription medications. Again, make sure you have your doctors' approval before taking any supplements to avoid any contraindications from medicines you are taking or conditions you have.

- *A comprehensive digestive enzyme.*

  The body may need help digesting carbohydrates, protein and fat as well as help balancing metabolism during weight loss. Digestive enzymes should be taken temporarily while you are losing the weight if you are under the age of 40; otherwise, a dependency could occur. Following your food plan well will help the body once again produce the enzymes adequately on its own. After the age of 40, a digestive enzyme may be necessary for continued optimal health as normal enzyme function depletes as we age. If you are Linked Type B, your digestive enzyme should contain enzymes to assist with proteins such as protease; enzymes to help with fats such as lipase; enzymes to help with carbohydrates such as amylase; and ox bile or bile salts to help support liver and gall bladder function.

- *A super food or super supplement.*
Herbal support such as Dandelion, Milk Thistle or Peppermint may be helpful for Linked Type B. These herbs can be taken as a supplement according to instructions on the label or in herbal tea form as often as you like. These herbs assist in healthy liver and gall bladder function, which is often a weak area for Linked Type B individuals.

Linked TYPE B Sample Meal Plan

	BREAKFAST (Fruit)	LUNCH (Main meal)	SNACK (Protein & veggie)	DINNER (Light meal)
SUN	Morning Tonic ¼ c blueberries, ¼ c strawberries, 1 banana Top with ½ c raw or slivered almonds.	1 c steamed broccoli ½ c cooked yellow lentils with fresh garlic and ginger ½ c brown rice 1 c kale stir-fried	1 c carrot juice 1 avocado ½ c almonds	Mixed-greens with: 1 shredded carrot ¼ c sliced almonds 2 oz wild salmon baked drizzle extra-virgin olive oil & ¼ lemon squeezed
MON	Morning Tonic ½ c blackberries ½ c blueberries 1 c tea with 2 TB almond milk	1 cooked turkey breast 1 c wilted spinach, ½ c sliced cucumber, 1 shredded carrot toss in extra-virgin olive oil & sea salt	1 c carrot juice 1 avocado ½ c cashews	Smoothie in blender: ½ c almond milk, 2 TB almond butter, 2 TB unsweetened cocoa powder, ¼ c raw cashews
TUES	Morning Tonic 1 baked apple cored & stuffed with chopped pecans with cinnamon 1 c chamomile tea	1 Tilapia sautéed in coconut oil 1 cucumber, sliced 1 avocado, sliced ½ c steamed broccoli	2 stalks of celery washed and cut into pieces, served with almond butter	1 large baked sweet potato drizzled with extra-virgin olive oil and sprinkled with sea salt
WED	Morning Tonic 2 TB almond butter with 1 apple or pear ½ c blueberries 1 c green tea with ½ tsp raw honey	1 c basmati or brown rice ½ c black beans 1 avocado 1 TB chopped tomato mixed w/ extra-virgin olive oil and sea salt	2 oz Goat cheese 1 raw pear, nectarine or peach	Homemade vegetable juice: 4-5 carrots ¼ of a beet 1 apple
THURS	Morning Tonic Mix ½ c gluten-free oatmeal, 1 TB flax meal, 1 TB unsweetened apple sauce ½ tsp cinnamon	4 large shrimp sautéed in extra-virgin olive oil, served with stir-fry of 2 T onion, 1 zucchini and 1 red bell pepper	1 banana sliced with ¼ c unsweetened almond milk poured over	Smoothie in blender: ½ c unsweetened almond milk, ½ c frozen/fresh strawberries, 2 TB almond butter
FRI	Morning Tonic Smoothie in blender: ½ c almond milk 2 TB almond butter 2 TB unsweetened cocoa powder, ¼ c raw cashews	1 Turkey burger wrapped in lettuce with 1 avocado 1 c side salad of mixed greens	1 apple with 2 TB almond butter	2-egg omelet with 1 sliced red bell pepper and ¼ c spinach
SAT	Fruit bowl: 1 apple, ½ c blueberries, ½ c strawberries, ½ c diced pineapple 1 c chamomile tea	1 c brown rice ½ c yellow lentils 1 c spinach with chopped mushrooms and red onion	1 c carrot juice 1 avocado ¼ c almonds	1 c blackberries with ¼ c coconut cream poured over

101

Linked Type B Breakfast Recipes

Apple Walnut Cream

Ingredients:
1 Gala apple
¼ cup raw walnuts
1 cup raw cashews
1 cups filtered water, divided
½ teaspoon vanilla extract

In a medium bowl, soak cashews in 1 cup or more, if needed, of filtered water for 4 hours. Drain and rinse. In a food processor, blend cashews, ½ cup filtered water and vanilla extract until creamy and smooth. Add more water if needed slowly, a little at a time until creamy consistency is reached.

Slice apple and lay on plate. Chop walnuts and sprinkle over apple. Spoon cashew cream on top of apple walnut mixture.

Refrigerate remaining cashew cream for later.

Blueberry Quinoa Pudding

Ingredients:
1 cup filtered water
½ cup uncooked quinoa
1 cup blueberries
1 cup unsweetened apple sauce
¼ teaspoon cinnamon

Bring water and quinoa to a boil in a small saucepan. Boil for 1–2 minutes and remove from heat. Cover and let sit until water is absorbed. Add blueberries, apple sauce and cinnamon. Mix well and press down into glass pan. Sprinkle with extra cinnamon, if desired.

Serve immediately or refrigerate and serve cold.

Hot Cereal

Ingredients:
2 cups filtered water
1 cup rolled oats
¼ cup chopped or slivered almonds
¼ cup raw sunflower seeds
1 Red Delicious apple
1 Bartlett pear
Cinnamon, for garnish (optional)

In a small saucepan, bring filtered water to a boil. Add oats and cook on reduced heat for 5-10 minutes until water is absorbed and oats have desired consistency. Remove from heat. Add almonds and sunflower seeds.

Peel, core and shred both apple and pear. In a separate bowl, mix fruits together.

Serve oatmeal with desired amount of fruit mixture spooned on top. Sprinkle with cinnamon.

Green Smoothie

Ingredients:
½ cup unsweetened almond milk
½ cup frozen berries
2 fresh spinach leaves
1 teaspoon raw honey
½ cup ice

Place all ingredients in a blender and blend until smooth and creamy.

Serve and drink immediately.

Veggie Omelet

Ingredients:
2 cage-free eggs
1 green onion, diced
½ red bell pepper, diced

1 avocado
1 tablespoon extra-virgin olive oil

Beat eggs in a small mixing bowl. Add green onion and red bell pepper. In a medium skillet, heat olive oil on medium heat. Move pan around to coat entire pan. Pour egg mixture into pan. Cover and cook until egg is cooked in the center. Slice avocado.

Serve avocado slices on top of omelet.

Tropical Fruit Salad

Ingredients:
1 cup pineapple, diced
½ cup unsweetened coconut flakes
1 ripe mango, sliced
1 peach, diced (1 banana on allowed days)
2 tablespoons unsweetened almond milk

In a medium bowl, add fruit and pour almond milk over top. Toss gently and serve.

Linked Type B Lunch Recipes

Turkey and Lentils

Ingredients:
3 cups filtered water
1 cup red or yellow lentils, uncooked
2 tablespoons olive oil
1 (2 to 4-ounce) turkey breast portion
1 stalk of celery, diced
½ cup white onion, diced
1 apple
Sea salt
Pepper

In small saucepan, bring filtered water and lentils to a boil. Simmer on medium heat for 10 minutes. Reduce heat to low until water is absorbed and lentils are tender.

In a skillet, heat olive oil on medium heat. Add diced onion and celery. Sprinkle with salt and pepper. Sauté 10 minutes or until tender. Slice turkey breast and add to skillet. Sauté until turkey is cooked thoroughly. Core and dice apple. Add to skillet. Cook additional 5-10 minutes.

Serve turkey mix over lentils.

Stuffed Peppers

Ingredients:
1 onion, diced
2 carrots, grated
1 fennel bulb, thinly sliced
1 cup celery, diced
2 green bell peppers
3 tablespoons extra-virgin olive oil
4 tablespoons tomato paste

Preheat oven to 350°F. In a large skillet, heat olive oil on medium heat. Add onion, carrots, fennel and celery. Cook 8–10 minutes or until vegetables are tender. Add tomato paste and stir.

Meanwhile, slice peppers in half and remove seeds. Lay flat in glass baking pan. Spoon veggie mixture into each half. Pour any liquid over the top. Cover with lid or foil and bake for 25-30 minutes.

Quinoa Mushroom Bake

Ingredients:
1 cup quinoa, uncooked
1 cup button or Crimini mushrooms, diced
2 shallots
1 clove of garlic, mined
1 carrot, shredded
1 cup chopped Swiss chard
2 cups vegetable broth
3 tablespoons extra-virgin olive oil
Sea salt
Pepper

Preheat oven to 325°F. In a medium saucepan, bring vegetable broth and quinoa to a boil. Boil for 5 minutes and remove from heat. Cover and let sit until broth is absorbed.

In a large skillet, heat oil on medium heat. Add garlic and shallots. Cook a few minutes until shallots are tender. Add mushrooms and cook until moisture from mushroom is absorbed. Add carrot and chard. Cook for a few minutes.

In a greased casserole pan, place veggies evenly on bottom. Scoop cooked quinoa and spread on top of veggies. Brush quinoa with olive oil and sprinkle with sea salt and pepper. Bake uncovered for 15-20 minutes or until quinoa has a golden shine.

Turkey Hot Pot

Ingredients:
4 turkey sausage links
½ head of green cabbage, diced
5 fingerling potatoes, shredded
½ onion, diced
6 tablespoons extra-virgin olive oil

In a large skillet, heat oil on medium heat. Shred potatoes and add to hot oil. Avoid overheating olive oil. Add onion and cabbage. Cook until shredded potato and cabbage are tender.

Remove casing from turkey sausage. Discard casing. In a separate skillet, break up turkey sausage and cook until brown. Add cooked turkey to potato mixture. Serve.

Vegetable Soup

Ingredients:
1 onion, diced
2 carrots, sliced
3 celery stalks, sliced
4 fingerling potatoes, diced very small
5 cloves garlic, minced
6 tablespoons olive oil
1 quart vegetable stock or broth
1 quart filtered water
1 cup arugula

In a large stock pot, heat olive oil on medium heat. Add minced garlic. Cook for a couple of minutes. Add diced onion. Cook until onion is caramelized (golden brown). Add carrots and celery and continue to cook for 5-10 minutes more. Add fingerling potatoes, stock and filtered water. Cook on medium heat for 15-20 minutes or until potatoes are fork-tender. Take off heat. Stir in arugula.

Serve immediately. Store remainder of soup in air-tight container for later.

Fish Hot Pot

Ingredients:
1 fish filet (cod, halibut or other meaty fish)
2 carrots
3 stalks of celery
1 yellow onion
½ red onion
1 red bell pepper
2 cups vegetable broth
3 tablespoons olive oil
Sea salt
Pepper

In large stock pot, heat oil on medium heat. Cut yellow and red onions into large chunks. Add onions and sprinkle generously with salt and pepper. Simmer for 5-10 minutes. Cut carrots, red bell pepper and celery into large chunks and add to pot. Add vegetable stock. Add fish in broken chunks. Cook until fish is thoroughly cooked. Toss frequently to mix flavors. Serve hot.

Linked Type B Dinner Recipes

Baked Potato with Arugula Salad

Ingredients:
1 quart water
1 yellow or red potato
2 tablespoons goat feta cheese
1 cups arugula
1 cup butter lettuce, chopped
1 Bartlett pear

¼ red onion
1 tablespoon extra-virgin olive oil
½ teaspoon mustard

Preheat oven to 350°F. In a medium sauce pan, bring water to a boil. Add potato. Keep water at a boil 10-20 minutes until potato is soft, and you can pierce a knife through it. Remove from water. Halve potato. Scoop out the insides and set aside in a small mixing bowl.

Add feta cheese to the potato insides and mix well. Spoon mixture back into potato skin halves and bake for 10-12 minutes. Meanwhile, slice pear very thin. Slice red onion into very thin strips. Mix oil and mustard in a small bowl. In a large bowl, add arugula and lettuce. Toss with mustard dressing. Add pear and onion. Toss again.

Serve baked potato with cold salad on the side.

Mediterranean Salad

Ingredients:
1 handful of fresh green beans
1 heart of romaine
1 yellow potato (optional)
1 egg, hard-boiled
2 Grape tomatoes (yellow and/or red)
3 Anchovy fillets
1 lemon

Prepare hard-boiled egg in advance: Place egg in water in sauce pot and bring to a boil. Boil for 10 minutes and remove egg from water. Rinse under cold water. Chill overnight, if able.

In a small saucepan, cover potato with water and bring to a boil. Boil for 10-15 minutes or until potato is cooked. Remove from water. Cut into large chunks. Set aside. In medium saucepan, bring a pot of water to boil. Add green beans for a quick 3–5 minutes to blanch. Drain and rinse with cold water.

On a large plate, arrange romaine lettuce and layer green beans and potato evenly on top. Slice hard-boiled egg. Arrange on top of potato. Quarter tomatoes and arrange. Place anchovy fillets on top. Drizzle with extra-virgin olive oil and squeeze a touch of fresh lemon around.

Serve immediately.

Mussels and Leeks

Ingredients:
1 bag of fresh mussels
2 stalks of leeks
3 cloves garlic, minced
1 cup vegetable broth
2 tablespoons olive oil
1 bunch fresh spinach
Sea salt

Wash mussels under running water. Discard any that are open. Set aside remaining mussels. In a large stock pot, simmer minced garlic in broth for 1-2 minutes. Add mussels and cover. Bring to a vigorous steam for about 10 minutes. Open to see if shells have opened. If they have, remove from heat. If not, cover and cook for another 5 minutes. Check again. Set aside.

In a small skillet, heat olive oil on medium heat. Wash leeks well to remove soil. Slice leeks. Add to skillet and sauté. Sprinkle with salt.

Wash spinach and arrange on a plate. Place sautéed leeks over spinach and a handful of cooked mussels on top. Serve. (Mussels are to be removed from the shell and eaten.)

Roasted Beets with Feta

Ingredients:
2 red beets with tops
3 tablespoons extra-virgin olive oil
1 tablespoon rice vinegar
¼ teaspoon mustard powder
¼ teaspoon dried parsley
¼ cup goat feta cheese

Preheat oven to 425°F. Wash beets, remove tops and peel. Quarter each beet and divide each quarter again. In a casserole baking pan, arrange beets face up. Place in oven uncovered and roast for 40-45 minutes or until fork-tender.

In a small bowl, mix oil, vinegar, mustard and parsley. When beets are cooked arrange in a large bowl. Toss with dressing and crumbled feta.

Serve warm.

Baked, Stuffed Sweet Potato

Ingredients:
1 large sweet potato
1 egg
Pinch of sea salt
Pinch of black pepper

Preheat oven to 375°F. Lay potato on baking sheet and bake 30–40 minutes until potato can be pierced with knife cleanly. Remove from oven.

Beat egg, salt and pepper in a small mixing bowl. Halve sweet potato lengthwise. Scoop out insides of each half. Place insides of the potato into the egg mixture. Mix well. Spoon mixture into potato skin halves. Place potato halves on baking sheet. Bake for another 10-15 minutes.

Serve immediately.

Linked TYPE C Food List and Supplements

60% of food	*40% of food*	*NOT AT ALL*
Fruit: ALL *Vegetables:* ALL especially Dark leafy greens (Spinach, arugula, kale, chard, turnip greens, etc.) *Nuts:* Almonds *Grains/Starches:* Fingerling potatoes Acorn, Butternut and Spaghetti Squash *Other:* Flax and Flax oil Extra-virgin Olive Oil Coconut and coconut oil (if tolerated well)	*Dairy:* Cage-free/organic eggs (pasture-fed is ideal) *Seafood:* Shrimp, Mussels Wild Salmon and Fish *Meats:* Organic chicken Turkey and Lamb *Nuts:* Pistachio, Walnuts Cashews and Hazelnuts *Grains/Starches:* Sweet potatoes White, red or yellow potatoes *Other:* Raw honey Organic butter Organic yogurt	*Fruit/Vegetables:* Produce imported from non-European countries *Grains/Starches:* Oats Enriched or white rice Gluten (no wheat or white flour foods) *Nuts:* Peanuts *Dairy:* Cow dairy (cheese, ice cream, sour cream, cream cheese) *Meats:* Pork (ham, bacon, pork chops, pork loin, etc.) Lobster Crab Tuna *Other:* Pinto and Kidney beans Corn (and corn oil) Canola oil Soy beans and soybean oil Hydrogenated and partially hydrogenated oils White and brown sugar, Aspartame, NutraSweet, Equal, Sweet n Low, Splenda High fructose corn syrup, Dextrose, Maltodextrin Dough conditioners

One time per week
AT MOST once every 4 days

Fruit/Vegetables: Raisins Peas *Grains/Starches:* Brown or Basmati rice *Meats:* Red meat (beef/buffalo) Chicken (cage-free or range-free, avoid regular chicken altogether)	*Dairy:* Goat products (goat feta, goat yogurt, goat milk) Organic cheese (from cow's milk) *Other:* Black, Navy and Lima beans Lentils Coconut and coconut oil Agave nectar Pure maple syrup

Guidelines to Increase Your Body's Response:

- Begin each day, 20 minutes before having breakfast, with this morning tonic: 8 ounces of water with 2 ounces of aloe vera juice and liquid chlorophyll (follow label recommendations for a single serving on the brand you purchase), a pinch of pink Himalayan sea salt, and one-half of a lemon-freshly squeezed.
- Breakfast must contain protein such as eggs or fish or almonds or yogurt.
- Make sure each of your main meals contains a significant protein source.
- Cook with herbs and spices such as garlic, lemon, pink Himalayan sea salt.

Supplement Considerations for Linked Type C

Supplements are key components of your Linked Diet. Foundational supplements, like multivitamins and minerals, are essential to maintain healthy nutritional levels and are intended for life-long use. Clean and repair supplements are NOT intended to be life-long supplements. Instead, they work to more quickly restore nutritional deficiencies that, without supplementation, may slowly and eventually disappear as proper foods are eaten consistently (resulting in the digestive changes needed to restore balance to the body.)

The best way to ensure you are getting the correct supplements that coincide with your Linked Type and your biochemical individuality is to consult with a nutritionist or other healthcare professional that specializes in this area. And remember, it is always a good idea to have your doctor's approval before making any dietary changes or taking any supplements to avoid any complications or unknown contraindications with medications. Please note supplement recommendations are not approved for women who are pregnant or nursing, adults who are taking prescription medications, or minors under the age of 18.

Consider the following supplements to enhance your Linked Type C food protocol:

- *A good multivitamin and mineral supplement.*
  A basic multivitamin may not have minerals. Read the label to make sure your multivitamin also contains these important minerals: calcium, magnesium, potassium, phosphorus, iodine, zinc, and selenium. Minerals are as equally important in a well-rounded supplement as vitamins.
- *An amino acid supplement.*
  Make sure this supplement contains all amino acids and not just a few. Amino acids may influence your energy, your sleep, your mood and emotional wellbeing. A protein powder is not the same thing as an amino acid supplement and should not be used as a replacement for amino acid in supplemental form.

- *A fish oil supplement.*

  Fish oil helps not only brain function but also intestinal function and repair. Linked Type C persons may suffer from a breakdown in the hair-like fibers (*villi*) in the small intestine and may need to address this deficiency with food and specific supplements such as fish oil, a probiotic and enzymes.

- *A probiotic with at least eight strains of bacteria that cumulatively account for over one billion organisms.*

  A high-potency probiotic is absolutely essential and foundational for everyone from infants to seniors and should be taken permanently. A probiotic should have at least eight different strains of bacteria, and total of over one billion organisms. Probiotics contain live, helpful bacteria and many require refrigeration. Only buy probiotics from companies or health care professionals that guarantee the potency.

- *Betaine HCL (with or without pepsin).*

  Linked Type C persons may very well have depleted stomach acid which may cause low appetite in the morning, trouble taking supplements without feeling nausea, occasional to frequent heartburn, and constipation. Low stomach acid will also decrease protein absorption causing a deficiency in amino acids. *If you have a history of ulcers, you should avoid taking this supplement. If you experience heartburn while taking Betaine HCL consult a practitioner familiar with dosing Betaine HCL.*

- *A comprehensive digestive enzyme supplement.*

  The body may need help digesting carbohydrates, protein and fat as well as help balancing metabolism during weight loss. Digestive enzymes should be taken temporarily while you are losing the weight if you are under the age of 40; otherwise, a dependency could occur. Following your food plan well will help the body once again produce enzymes adequately on its own. After the age of 40, a digestive enzyme may be necessary for continued optimal health as normal enzyme function depletes as we age. If you are Linked Type C, your digestive enzyme should contain enzymes to assist with proteins such as protease; enzymes to help with fats such as lipase; and enzymes to help with carbohydrates such as amylase. A word of caution for Linked Type C digestive enzymes: avoid digestive enzymes already containing Betaine HCL since it is recommended that you take this supplement alone.

- *Super foods or super supplement.*

  Consider taking aloe vera juice, which will act as a great restorer to the digestive tract. This juice helps soothe the stomach lining and intestinal membranes and may have a truly positive affect on your weight. Aloe vera juice can be taken as the label recommends.

Linked TYPE C Sample Meal Plan

	BREAKFAST (Protein)	LUNCH (Protein & veggie)	SNACK (Protein & veggie)	DINNER (Light meal)
SUN	Morning Tonic ¼ c blueberries, ¼ c strawberries, ¼ c slivered almonds over 1 c plain organic yogurt	1 c steamed broccoli 2 oz smoked or baked salmon Sliced mango	1 c carrot juice 1 avocado ½ c almonds	Mixed-greens salad with:1 shredded carrot ¼ c sliced almonds, Hardboiled egg. Extra-virgin olive oil and squeeze ¼ lemon
MON	Morning Tonic 1 to 2-egg omelet with spinach and red bell pepper 1 c herbal tea	1 cooked Turkey breast. Salad with: 1 c spinach, ½ c sliced cucumber, shredded carrot. Toss w extra-virgin olive oil & sea salt	1 c unsweetened apple sauce ½ c cashews	Smoothie in blender: ½ c almond milk 2 TB almond butter 2 TB unsweetened cocoa powder ¼ c raw cashews
TUES	Morning Tonic Smoothie in blender: ½ c almond milk 1 banana 1 c frozen mango ½ c ice	1 chicken breast sautéed in coconut oil 1 cucumber, sliced 1 avocado, sliced 1 Roma tomato with extra-virgin olive oil	2 stalks of celery washed and cut into pieces with almond butter	1 large baked sweet potato drizzled with extra-virgin olive oil and sprinkled with sea salt
WED	Morning Tonic 1 c plain organic yogurt ½ c strawberries ½ c slivered almonds	2 shredded fingerling potatoes mixed with 1 beaten egg, fried in coconut oil, served over spinach.	2 oz Goat cheese 1 raw pear, nectarine or peach	Homemade vegetable juice: 4-5 carrots ¼ of a beet 1 apple
THUR	Morning Tonic 1-2 turkey sausage sliced avocado and sliced apple	4 large shrimp sautéed in extra virgin olive oil Stir-fry: 2 TB onion, 1 zucchini and 1 red bell pepper	1 banana sliced with ¼ c unsweetened almond milk poured over	Smoothie in blender: ½ c unsweetened almond milk, ½ c frozen or fresh strawberries, 2 TB almond butter
FRI	Morning Tonic Smoothie in blender: ½ c unsweetened almond milk 2 TB almond butter 2 TB unsweetened cocoa powder ¼ c raw cashews	1 turkey burger wrapped in lettuce with 1 avocado 1 c side salad of mixed greens	1 apple with 2 TB almond butter	2 egg omelet with 1 sliced red bell pepper and ¼ c spinach
SAT	1 banana sliced with almond milk poured over the top, sprinkled with cinnamon 1 c chamomile tea	1 c brown rice ½ c yellow lentils 1 c spinach with chopped mushrooms and red onion	1 c carrot juice 1 avocado ¼ c almonds	1 c blackberries with ¼ c coconut cream poured over

Linked Type C Breakfast Recipes

Yogurt Parfait

Ingredients:
1 cup plain organic yogurt
½ cup blueberries or strawberries
¼ cup chopped hazelnuts (or slivered almonds)
1 tablespoon pure maple syrup

Place yogurt in a small bowl, then place berries on top. Sprinkle with nuts. Top with drizzled maple syrup.

Smoked Salmon Omelet

Ingredients:
2 cage-free eggs
3 ounces smoked salmon
4 green onions, chopped (or 2 tablespoon chives)
1 tablespoon organic butter
2 tablespoons plain yogurt

Heat butter in a small skillet, moving it around to grease bottom of skillet. Beat eggs in a small bowl and slowly pour eggs into skillet. Cover and cook on a low heat until egg is cooked. Slide egg out of skillet onto plate. Place salmon and chopped green onions on one side of egg. Fold egg over onto salmon. Dollop yogurt on top. Serve.

Eggs and Hash

Ingredients:
3 fingerling potatoes
4 tablespoons organic butter
¼ yellow onion, diced
5 eggs, divided
1 teaspoon fresh or dried rosemary
Sea salt
Pepper

Shred potatoes into a bowl. Set aside. In a small skillet, heat butter. Add yellow onion. Open one egg into a small bowl. Separate remaining egg, adding yolk to other egg and egg white to potatoes.

Mix egg white and potatoes well. Add potato mixture to hot skillet. Cover and allow to brown on one side. Flip potatoes. (Do not worry if potato breaks apart.) Sprinkle with rosemary. Season with salt and pepper to taste. Move potatoes from pan to plate.

Pour remaining egg into pan without beating. Cook egg sunny-side-up. Remove when egg is cooked and slide on top of potato hash.

Serve immediately.

Hearty Tropical Salad

Ingredients:
1 banana, sliced
1 cup pineapple, diced
½ cup coconut flakes
2 tablespoons raisins
3 tablespoons chopped macadamia nuts (or hazelnuts)
¼ cup coconut milk (or cream)
¼ teaspoon cinnamon

Toss first 5 ingredients together in a small mixing bowl. Pour coconut milk over the top. Sprinkle with cinnamon. Serve.

Apple Cinnamon Muffins

Ingredients:
4 bananas
5 eggs
½ cup unsweetened applesauce
¼ cup olive oil
1 teaspoon vanilla
½ cup crunchy almond butter
¼ cup almond meal
½ teaspoon baking soda
½ teaspoon baking powder

¼ teaspoon sea salt
½ cup dried apricots, chopped

Preheat oven to 325°F. In a blender, blend banana, eggs, applesauce, oil and vanilla until all is smooth. Add almond butter and blend. Pour into bowl and set aside. In a large mixing bowl, mix almond meal, baking soda, baking powder and sea salt. Mix well. Add banana mixture. Mix well. Fold in dried apricots.

Place paper or foil liners in muffin cups. Pour almost a ¼ cup batter into each muffin cup. Bake 15-20 minutes or until cooked. (Test muffins by placing a knife, toothpick or cake tester in the center and see if it comes out clean.)

Linked Type C Lunch Recipes

Stuffed Avocado

Ingredients:
2 ounces small deveined shrimp or chicken breast, already cooked
1 avocados
1 tablespoon lemon juice
1 tablespoon olive oil
1 tablespoon salsa
Sea salt
Pepper

Chop cooked shrimp or chicken meat into small pieces and place in a small bowl. Add lemon juice and olive oil. Add sea salt and pepper to taste. Halve avocados and remove pits. Spoon mixture evenly into the avocados. Top with salsa. Serve.

Ginger Chicken and Carrots

Ingredients:
2 ounces organic chicken breast
3 green onions
4 carrots, shredded
1 cup lacinato kale
1 tablespoon fresh ginger, grated

1 tablespoon coconut or olive oil
Sea salt
Pepper

Slice chicken breast into thin strips. Chop green onion into large chunks. Shred carrots. Chop or slice kale. In a medium skillet, heat oil. Add green onion and ginger. Sprinkle with sea salt and pepper. Cook until golden or translucent. Add chicken and cook until chicken is thoroughly cooked. Add carrots. Cook for a few minutes. Add kale. Cook for only 1 minute, leaving green onions slightly crisp. Serve.

Substitute with other types of allowable meat/protein if needed such as fish, shrimp or turkey.

Buffalo Burger and Fries

Ingredients:
2 ounces ground buffalo
¼ teaspoon sea salt
¼ teaspoon black pepper
1 zucchini
2 tablespoons diced red onion
3 tablespoons coconut oil or olive oil, divided

In a mixing bowl, add ground buffalo, salt, pepper and 1 tablespoon of oil. Blend well. Shape buffalo mixture into burger size patties. Set aside.

Cut zucchini into french fries. Lay zucchini in one layer on baking sheet and sprinkle with salt. Let sit for 5-10 minutes until zucchini "sweats" moisture. Rinse quickly with water and pat dry. In a large skillet, heat remaining oil, then place zucchini fries evenly in pan. Remove from pan when golden on one side. Keep warm.

Place buffalo patties in hot skillet used for zucchini fries. Cook on one side and flip and cook other side. Continue to cook to desired doneness.

Serve with zucchini fries.

Chicken Waldorf Salad

Ingredients:
4 ounces cooked chicken breast
1 Gala apple
½ cup seedless green grapes
1 celery stalk
¼ cup chopped almonds or chopped walnuts
1 tablespoon extra-virgin olive oil
1 teaspoon mustard

Core apple and cut into bite size chunks. Slice grapes in half. Chop celery into very small pieces. Chop cooked chicken breast into small pieces. Combine all ingredients in a medium mixing bowl and stir well. Serve.

HINT: If chicken is uncooked, cook chicken thoroughly. Then, you can plunge chicken into ice water to quick-chill it for the salad; or you can make a warm salad using freshly cooked chicken.

Cauliflower Crunch Salad

Ingredients:
1 head cauliflower
1 bunch fresh parsley
1 Roma tomato (optional)
1 tablespoon lemon juice
1 tablespoon olive oil

In a large skillet, grate the cauliflower tops into the skillet and discard the stems of the cauliflower. Stir the contents of the skillet constantly. Cook for only 2 minutes. Set aside. Chop parsley into small pieces. Chop tomato into large pieces. In a medium mixing bowl, toss all ingredients together blending olive oil and lemon juice. Serve. Can substitute with radish on days tomatoes are not allowed.

Greek Salad

Ingredients:
1 head of Romaine lettuce
¼ cup Kalamata olives, pitted
¼ cup goat feta cheese

2 Roma tomatoes
1 cucumber
1 tablespoon olive oil
Sea salt

Chop lettuce, olives, and tomato into small pieces. Peel, if desired, and chop cucumber into small pieces. In a mixing bowl, combine all vegetable ingredients. Crumble feta over the top. Drizzle olive oil. Sprinkle with sea salt. Toss and serve.

Linked Type C Dinner Recipes

Turkey and Vegetables

Ingredients:
1 tablespoon olive oil
1 turkey cutlets (or breast meat)
1 red bell pepper
1 head of broccoli
1 carrot, shredded
1 sprig of fresh basil, chopped
½ cup chicken or vegetable broth
1 small can of coconut milk
1 sprig of fresh parsley, chopped
Pinch of cayenne pepper (optional)

In a large skillet, heat olive oil to a moderate temperature. Add turkey cutlet. Brown on both sides until cooked through. Remove from heat. Slice turkey into thin strips.

Meanwhile, seed bell pepper and cut into large chunks. Cut off and discard broccoli stems. Chop broccoli flowerettes into bite-size pieces. Chop basil and parsley.

Once turkey is removed from pan, stir-fry vegetables and herbs in pan for 2-4 minutes or until vegetables are tender but not too soft and overcooked. (Add additional oil if needed.) Add broth and turkey. Stir in ¼ cup coconut milk. Add cayenne. Cook for approximately 5 more minutes until heated through. If needed, continue to stir in small amounts coconut milk until desired consistency is reached.

Southwest Chicken Soup

Ingredients:
1 chicken breast
1 yellow onion
1 garlic clove
1 small can of diced green chiles
1 small can of diced tomatoes
1 carrot, shredded
1 quart chicken broth or vegetable broth
¼ teaspoon sea salt
¼ teaspoon black pepper
1 tablespoon coconut oil (or olive oil)

Heat oil in a large stock pot. Peel and dice yellow onion. Peel and mince garlic. Add yellow onion and garlic to pot. Cut chicken into bite-size pieces and add to pot. Add shredded carrot. Add remaining ingredients. Simmer until chicken is fully cooked, approximately 10–12 minutes.

Warm Spinach Salad with Goat Cheese

Ingredients:
2 cups fresh spinach leaves
¼ cup red onion
¼ cup goat feta cheese
1 cup Crimini mushrooms, sliced
1 tablespoon olive oil
Sea salt

Heat oil in a small skillet. Add sliced mushrooms and sprinkle with salt. While mushrooms are cooking, wash spinach and chop if necessary. Arrange spinach on plate. Peel and slice onion very thinly and place on top spinach. When mushrooms are cooked and while still hot, spoon mushrooms over spinach. Crumble feta on top.

Serve immediately.

Egg and Lemon Soup

Ingredients:
1 quart of chicken broth or vegetable broth
¼ cup Basmati rice
2 cage-free eggs
¼ cup fresh lemon juice (approximately 4 lemons)
Up to 1 quart filtered water (optional)

In a medium to large stock pot, bring chicken broth to a boil. Add rice. Reduce heat and simmer until rice is tender. (Add up to 1 quart filtered water if soup is too thick after rice is cooked.) Beat eggs in a bowl and very, very slowly pour the beaten eggs into hot broth. Egg will cook instantly into ribbons. Continue to cook for a few minutes. Add lemon juice.

Serve immediately.

Cod and Vegetables

Ingredients:
3 fingerling potatoes, sliced
4 carrots, sliced
1 celery stalk, sliced
1 garlic clove, minced
1 cod fillet
1 sprig of parsley
1 cup chicken or vegetable broth
2 tablespoons olive oil
½ cup coconut milk (optional)

In a medium stock pot, heat the broth. Add sliced vegetables and minced garlic. Slow simmer until vegetables are tender. Meanwhile, in a small skillet, heat olive oil. Add cod and brown on each side. Cod is fully cooked when the fish flakes when tested in the middle. Remove from heat. Cut into pieces and fold cod into vegetables. Drizzle with coconut milk over top. Toss altogether.

Serve immediately.

Linked TYPE D Food List and Supplements

80% of food	*20% of food*	*NOT AT ALL*
Fruit: ALL (except bananas, grapes, mangoes and pomegranates) **Vegetables:** ALL (except peas) Dark leafy greens (spinach, arugula, kale, chard, turnip greens, etc.) **Nuts:** Almonds Raw cashews **Grains/Starches:** Acorn, Butternut and Spaghetti Squash Quinoa **Other:** Flax and Flax oil, Extra-virgin Olive Oil Coconut and coconut oil	**Dairy:** Cage-free/organic eggs (pasture-fed is ideal) **Seafood:** Shrimp, Mussels Wild Salmon and all other Fish **Meats:** Turkey Lamb **Nuts:** Pistachios Walnuts Pecans Hazelnuts **Other:** Lentils (yellow or red) Raw honey	**Fruit/Vegetables:** Bananas, grapes, mangoes, pomegranates, raisins and dates Fruit juices Tomatoes and Peas Produce imported from non-European countries **Starches:** Oats Potatoes and Sweet potatoes Brown and enriched/white rice Gluten (no wheat or white flour foods) **Dairy:** Cow dairy (cheese, milk, cream, yogurt, ice cream) **Meats:** Red meat (Beef or Buffalo), Pork (ham, bacon, chops, loin, etc.) Lobster, Crab, and Tuna **Other:** Peanuts Corn and corn oil Canola oil Soybean oil and organic soy beans Kidney and pinto beans Hydrogenated and partially hydrogenated oils Chewing gum White and brown sugar, Aspartame, NutraSweet, Equal, Sweet n Low, and Splenda High fructose corn syrup, Dextrose, and Maltodextrin Dough conditioners and MSG Autolyzed yeast and soy proteins Autloyzed yeast extract

One time per week
AT MOST once every 4 days

Fruit/Vegetables: Oranges **Meats:** Chicken (organic only)	**Dairy**: Goat products (goat feta, goat yogurt, goat milk) Organic butter (from cow's milk) **Other**: Black, Navy and Lima beans

Guidelines to Increase Your Body's Response:

- Begin each day, 20 minutes before having breakfast, with this morning tonic: 8 ounces of water with 2 ounces of aloe vera juice and liquid chlorophyll (follow label recommendations for a single serving on the brand you purchase), a pinch of pink Himalayan sea salt, and one-half of a lemon-freshly squeezed.
- Breakfast must contain protein such as eggs or fish or almonds with cleansing and low sugar fruit such as apple or pear or berries.
- Make sure each of your main meals contain significant source of vegetables.
- Cook with herbs and spices such as garlic, lemon, pink Himalayan sea salt.
- Consume 8 ounces of filtered water with 1 teaspoon of Bragg Apple Cider Vinegar between 3:00 pm and 5:00 pm daily.

Supplement Considerations for Linked Type D

Supplements are key components of your Linked Diet. Foundational supplements, like multivitamins and minerals, are essential to maintain healthy nutritional levels and are intended for life-long use. Clean and repair supplements are NOT intended to be life-long supplements. Instead, they work to more quickly restore nutritional deficiencies that, without supplementation, may slowly and eventually disappear as proper foods are eaten consistently (resulting in the digestive changes needed to restore balance to the body.)

The best way to ensure you are getting the correct supplements that coincide with your Linked Type and your biochemical individuality is to consult with a nutritionist or other healthcare professional that specializes in this area. And remember, it is always a good idea to have your doctor's approval before making any dietary changes or taking any supplements to avoid any complications or unknown contraindications with medications. Please note supplement recommendations are not approved for women who are pregnant or nursing, adults who are taking prescription medications, or minors under the age of 18.

Consider the following supplements to enhance your Linked Type D food protocol:

- *A good multivitamin and mineral supplement.*
  A basic multivitamin may not have minerals. Read the label to make sure your multivitamin also contains these important minerals: calcium, magnesium, potassium, phosphorus, iodine, zinc, and selenium. Minerals are as equally important in a well-rounded supplement as vitamins.
- *Extra magnesium paired with a multivitamin that has calcium*
  This may be an important piece to help move things along while restoring your digestive health. Extra magnesium in addition to a multivitamin and mineral supplement that

already contains calcium and magnesium can help you have daily bowel movements as well as improve bowel function and ease. If daily bowel movements are not happening, then weight loss can be stunted. Try an additional 100–200mg of magnesium glycinate or magnesium citrate every night before bed in addition to your multivitamin. The extra magnesium may or may not be needed after you lose the weight to keep your bowel movements regular. Be sure to eat plenty of good fruits and vegetables while taking the magnesium to get good fiber.

- *An amino acid supplement.*

Make sure this supplement contains all amino acids and not just a few. Amino acids may influence your energy, your sleep, your mood and emotional wellbeing. A protein powder is not the same thing as an amino acid supplement and should not be used as a replacement for amino acid in supplemental form.

- *A probiotic with at least eight strains of bacteria that cumulatively account for over one billion organisms.*

A high-potency probiotic is absolutely essential and foundational for everyone from infants to seniors and should be taken permanently. A probiotic should have at least eight different strains of bacteria, and total of over one billion organisms. Probiotics contain live, helpful bacteria and many require refrigeration. Only buy probiotics from companies or health care professionals that guarantee the potency.

- *Betaine HCL.*

Low appetite in the morning, trouble taking supplements without feeling nausea, and occasional to frequent heartburn and constipation are very likely due to depleted stomach acid in Linked Type D persons. This depletion occurs when there is a yeast overgrowth in the intestinal track, which diminishes nutrient absorption. Low stomach acid will also decrease protein absorption causing a deficiency in amino acids. *If you have a history of ulcers, you should avoid taking this supplement. If you experience heartburn while taking Betaine HCL consult a practitioner familiar with dosing Betaine HCL.*

- *A comprehensive digestive enzyme.*

The body may need help digesting carbohydrates, protein and fat as well as help balancing metabolism during weight loss. Digestive enzymes should be taken temporarily while you are losing the weight if you are under the age of 40; otherwise, a dependency could occur. Following your food plan well will help the body once again produce the enzymes adequately on its own. After the age of 40, a digestive enzyme may be necessary for continued optimal health as normal enzyme function depletes as we age. If you are Linked Type D, your digestive enzyme should contain enzymes to assist with proteins such as protease, enzymes to help with fats such as lipase; and enzymes to help with carbohydrates such as amylase.

- *An antifungal regime.*
  Linked Type D may have yeast or fungal overgrowth in the intestinal track making nutrient absorption and weight loss difficult without addressing yeast or Candida overgrowth. Yeast or Candida is often difficult to reduce back to normal levels when overgrowth happens because the organisms will often adapt and resist the antifungal. Linked Type D may benefit from a fiber supplement or fiber powder such as psyllium in combination with an antifungal such as Grapefruit Seed Extract, Berberine, or Caprylic Acid.

Linked TYPE D Sample Meal Plan

	BREAKFAST (Protein)	LUNCH (Protein & veggie)	SNACK (Protein & veggie/fruit)	DINNER (Light meal)
SUN	Morning Tonic Smoothie: ½ c almond milk, 2 TB almond butter ½ c frozen blueberries	1 c steamed broccoli 1 sliced cucumber 1 half avocado 2 oz turkey	2 T almond butter 1 apple	Carrots salad: 2 carrots shredded ½ c diced pineapple ¼ c chopped pecans 1 c diced jicama
MON	Morning Tonic Veggie omelet with 1-2 eggs, spinach and red bell pepper 1 c herbal tea	2 oz chicken breast ½ c sautéed celery (2 stalks cooked in coconut oil) Sliced apple	½ c raw cashews ½ blackberries	Simmer: 1 c diced tomatoes 1 small onion diced 1 minced garlic 1 green bell pepper, diced, 1 qt vegetable broth
TUES	Morning Tonic Smoothie: ½ c almond milk 1 c frozen peaches 3 kale leaves	1 tilapia pan-fried in coconut oil Serve over raw spinach and sliced tomatoes	2 stalks of celery washed and cut into pieces with almond butter	Greens beans simmered in olive oil. Served with slivered almonds on top.
WED	Morning Tonic 2 oz cooked or smoked salmon 1 avocado, sliced 1 Gala apple	Stir-fry: 2 oz sirloin, thinly sliced 1 zucchini sliced, 1 red bell pepper & ½ onion chopped	2 oz Goat cheese 1 raw pear	Acorn squash, baked and diced, with dried apricots and chopped walnuts poured over the top
THUR	Morning Tonic Frittata: 2 eggs, 2 TB clean salsa (no sugar) 1TB tapioca flour Mix and cook in muffin tin.	2 oz baked salmon Fresh spinach	Hardboiled egg ½ c baby carrots	Spinach Salad: spinach, red onion sliced thin, goat feta cheese and sliced pear
FRI	Morning Tonic Hardboiled egg raw cashews apple	Lettuce wrap with ground beef, or turkey, and shredded carrot	1 c unsweetened applesauce sprinkled with ½ c chopped hazelnuts or slivered almonds	Broccoli florets sautéed with 1 TB plum fruit spread ¼ c slivered almonds
SAT	Scrambled egg with fruit of choice	½ c yellow lentils 1 c spinach with chopped red onion	1 avocado 1 apple	1 c blackberries with ¼ c coconut cream poured over

Linked Type D Breakfast Recipes

Stuffed Crookneck

Ingredients:
1 yellow crookneck squash
2 teaspoons coconut oil, divided
1 turkey sausage link
1 egg, beaten
2 teaspoons coconut oil
1 tablespoon olive oil

Preheat oven to 425°F. Cut squash on long side to create two long halves. Scoop out seeds and discard. Brush 1 teaspoon of coconut oil on each half. Put into oven for 15 minutes.

Remove and discard casing from sausage. Place olive oil and sausage in a small skillet. Cook sausage until browned. Add beaten egg. Stir in beaten egg. Cook mixture until egg is cooked. When squash is done, scoop sausage mixture evenly into both halves. Serve.

Cream of Strawberry

Ingredients:
1 cup fresh strawberries, sliced
2 tablespoons chopped hazelnut or slivered almonds (optional)
½ cup canned coconut cream, chilled

Wash the strawberries. Slice and arrange in a bowl. Drizzle coconut cream over strawberries. Sprinkle with hazelnuts or other allowable nuts. Serve.

HINT: Keep canned coconut cream in the refrigerator until ready to use.

Watermelon Granata and Pears

Ingredients:
3 cups watermelon (1 small watermelon)
4 tablespoons fresh raspberry
1 Bartlett pear

2 tablespoons sliced almonds
¼ teaspoon cinnamon
½ cup ice

Seed, peel and cut up watermelon. Place watermelon in blender with raspberry and ice. Blend until smooth. Chill in freezer for 10-15 minutes. Pour watermelon mixture into bowl. Slice pear very thin. Arrange slices on top. Sprinkle with almonds. Dust with cinnamon. Serve.

Baked Walnut Apples

Ingredients:
1 apple
½ cup chopped walnuts
½ teaspoon cinnamon
¼ teaspoon nutmeg
1 teaspoon pure maple syrup

Preheat oven to 350°F. Core apple. Grease a baking pan. Place apple upright in pan. In a small bowl, mix walnuts, cinnamon, nutmeg and syrup. Stuff mixture into middle of apple. Bake for 20 minutes or until apple has desired tenderness.

Lox and Asparagus

Ingredients:
2 ounces salmon lox
1 tablespoon Chevrie˙ spreadable goat cheese
2 asparagus spears
1 tablespoon olive oil
1 fresh lemon

Spread lox open. Spread goat cheese onto lox. Place an asparagus spear in at one end. Roll lox around asparagus. Repeat for each remaining asparagus spear. Arrange on a plate. Drizzle the olive oil over spears. Squeeze a bit of lemon juice over top. Serve.

Linked Type D Lunch Recipes

Turkey Burger and Zucchini Salad

Ingredients:
1 zucchini
1 carrot
2 ounces ground turkey
3 tablespoons diced red onion
1 tablespoon coconut oil
¼ teaspoon sea salt
¼ teaspoon black pepper
1 tablespoon olive oil

Shred zucchini. Cut carrot julienne-style. Lay on a baking sheet and sprinkle with salt. Wait 10 minutes for vegetables to "sweat" extra moisture. Rinse and pat dry. Set on plate.

In a small bowl, mix turkey, onion, sea salt, black pepper, and coconut oil. Mix well with your hands and shape into a patty. In a small skillet, heat olive oil on a low heat. Place turkey burger in pan and cook until browned on one side. Flip and cook the other side.

Serve with the zucchini.

Quinoa Salad Greek Style

Ingredients:
½ cup uncooked quinoa
1 cup water
1 cucumber
2-3 small red radishes
4 or 5 pitted kalamata olives
1 bunch fresh parsley
2 tablespoons goat feta cheese
1 tablespoon olive oil
Pinch of sea salt

In a small stock pot, bring water and quinoa to a boil. Slow simmer until water is absorbed and quinoa is tender. If quinoa is too crunchy, you can add additional water, bring to a boil and reduce heat again until desired softness is obtained. Rinse the cooked quinoa in a tight weave strainer under cold water. Set aside.

Peel, seed and dice cucumber. Chop olives and slice the radishes. Chop parsley very small. In a bowl, toss quinoa, radishes, parsley, cucumber, klamata olives, goat feta, olive oil and sea salt. Mix well. Serve.

Shrimp Rolls

Ingredients:
Butter lettuce leaves (one for each roll being made)
1 cup of small, cooked peeled and deveined shrimp (prepared ahead and chilled)
1 carrot, shredded
Very thin red onion slices (one or two for each roll being made)
1 avocado, sliced

Take each lettuce leaf and add a spoonful of the cooked shrimp, some carrot, onion and one or two avocado slices. Roll lettuce around the mixture. Repeat process for each roll being made. Serve.

Black Bean Soup

Ingredients:
1 large can black beans, rinsed
1 quart chicken or vegetable stock or broth
2 large carrots, sliced
1 small yellow onion
1 tablespoon olive oil
Sea salt
Black pepper

In a medium stock pot, heat oil on moderate heat. Peel and dice onion. Add to pot. Slice the carrots and add to the pot. Sprinkle with sea salt and pepper. Simmer a few minutes until onion and carrot is tender. Add rinsed beans and the chicken or vegetable broth/stock. Simmer for a few minutes until thoroughly heated. Take half the mixture and puree in food processor. Stir puree back into pot. Serve.

Seafood Spinach Salad

Ingredients:
1 cup seafood, cooked (either shrimp, tilapia, cod or salmon)
2 cups spinach leaves (washed, stems removed)
1 orange bell pepper
1 yellow bell pepper
2 tablespoons olive oil
1 fresh lemon

Seed peppers and cut into chunks. Toss peppers with seafood, spinach, and olive oil. Toss well to mix oil. Drizzle fresh-squeezed lemon over salad. Serve.

Quick Broccoli Soup

Ingredients:
1 head of broccoli
1 quart of filtered water or vegetable broth
1 teaspoon sea salt
1 carrot

Cut off base of broccoli leaving a good amount of stem. Place entire head into a stock pot with 2 inches of water. Cover and bring water to a boil. Steam broccoli for 5 minutes or until broccoli is bright green and slightly tender, but not overcooked. Remove from heat and rinse with cool water for 1 minute. Place in food processor with enough filtered water for broccoli to puree. Pour into a stock pot and add remaining water. Add sea salt and bring to a simmer. Shred carrot.

Serve soup in bowl and sprinkle raw shredded carrot over the top.

Grilled Portabello and Spinach

Ingredients:
1 large portabello mushroom
2 shallots
1 garlic clove, minced
1 tablespoon olive oil
1 cup spinach leaves

Heat olive oil in a large skillet. Add garlic. Peel shallot and slice thin. Add to garlic and oil. Wash mushroom and snap off stem. Slice mushroom into thick slices and add to skillet. Sauté for 5 minutes. Turn off heat. Throw spinach into skillet and mix for 10 seconds and remove food from pan immediately.

Serve immediately.

Linked Type D Dinner Recipes

Spaghetti Squash Pesto

Ingredients:
1 small spaghetti squash
1 handful fresh basil
¼ cup pine nuts
¼ cup olive oil
¼ cup Pecorino Romano cheese (from sheep's milk)

Preheat oven to 350°F. Slice squash in half lengthwise and remove seeds. Place face down in baking pan with couple of inches of water. Bake for 30–40 minutes.

Shred Pecorino Romano cheese. In a food processor, add basil (stems removed), pine nuts, olive oil, and cheese. Process until a creamy pesto forms. When squash is finished baking, remove from oven. Scrape pulp out. Discard squash skins. Break pulp apart with fork forming spaghetti-like strands. Toss with pesto. Serve.

Unbelievably Good Lamb Chops

Ingredients:
2 lamb chops (can use extras for lunches)
3 yellow potatoes
4 tablespoons olive oil, divided
1 tablespoon yellow mustard
1 teaspoon sea salt
¼ teaspoon black pepper
1 cup arugula

Preheat oven to 325°F. In a pot, cover potatoes with water and bring to a boil. Boil for 15-10 minutes until potato is extra-tender when pierced. Drain and let cool. To cool quickly, rinse under cool water. Peel potatoes with your fingers. Place potatoes in bowl. Add 2 tablespoons olive oil and mash with a potato masher. Set aside and keep warm.

In a small bowl, add mustard, sea salt, pepper and remaining 2 tablespoons olive oil. Mix with fork. Spread mustard mixture on front and back of lamb chops. Place chops on baking sheet. Bake for 20–25 minutes or until fat on lamb is sizzling and the center of the chop is thoroughly cooked.

Place a handful of arugula on a plate. Spoon some mashed potato on top arugula. Serve lamb chop over mashed potato.

Dinner in a Glass

Ingredients:
½ cup ice
1 apple, peeled and cored
1 cup spinach, washed
½ blueberries
1 peach, stem removed
1 kale leaf
Filtered water (optional)

Place ice in a blender. Add all remaining ingredients. Blend until smooth. If mixture is too thick or will not blend, add small amount of filtered water at a time.

Serve immediately.

Leek and Potato Soup

Ingredients:
2 fingerling potatoes
1 white onion
2 leeks
3 shallots
4 cloves of garlic, minced

5 tablespoons olive oil
1 quart vegetable (or chicken) broth

Heat oil in a large stock pot. Peel and slice shallots. Add shallots and minced garlic to hot oil. Dice onion and add to pot. Wash leeks very well. Make sure hidden soil and dirt is washed away. Cut ends off and discard. Slice leeks very thin and add to pot. As leeks cook they break apart. Slice very thin or grate potatoes and add to pot. Add broth. Cook until potatoes are tender.

Serve as is or, for thicker consistency, puree half or all of mixture in blender or food processor until creamy before serving.

Flank Steak and Arugula

Ingredients:
2 ounces flank steak (or sirloin)
1 cup arugula
1 red (or orange) bell pepper
1 tablespoon coconut oil

Heat oil in a large skillet. Cook flank steak for 5-10 minutes on each side to desired doneness. Seed pepper and slice into thin strips. Add around meat. Turn as needed. After meat is cooked, remove from pan and use a sharp knife carefully and slice meat very thin.

Arrange arugula on a plate. Either lay meat with pepper on top arugula or lay meat on top arugula and arrange pepper around the meat. Serve.

Skillet Meat Sauce

Ingredients:
2 ounces ground turkey
1 tablespoon coconut oil
1 small can diced (or crushed) tomato
2 zucchini

Cut off ends of zucchini. Slice zucchini julienne-style avoiding seeds in center. Discard ends and seed middle. Lay zucchini on baking sheet and sprinkle with salt. Wait 10 minutes for zucchini to "sweat" extra moisture. Rinse and pat dry. Set aside.

In a skillet, heat oil and add ground turkey. Break apart and cook thoroughly. When turkey is done, add tomatoes and simmer.

Serve over raw zucchini "noodles."

ENDNOTES

You are now at the end of this book, but not the end of your journey. If you have been following the mindset steps and action steps while also following your personal Linked Type food plan, you are at least twenty-one days into your personal journey of connecting mindset, digestive health and weight loss to achieve your best self.

As you continue to move forward, here are some tips to help you continue on your journey. Keep up your efforts in your Linked Type food plan until you reach your weight goal. Keep up your mindset steps with a journal of your own. Make sure you continue with the daily exercises of gratitude, affirmations and reminding yourself of the things in your life that went well that particular day. A positive mindset on a daily basis is important for keeping an upward momentum and staying successful.

If you are interesting in fine-tuning your Linked Type into even more customization, please feel free to schedule an appointment with me at www.laurakopec.com. I consult with individuals by phone or in person, so it does not matter where you live. If you live outside Texas and want the personal touch of someone local to you, make sure you look for a practitioner or educator that specializes in functional imbalances and whole body wellness.

I welcome any feedback, comments or personal insights into your journey with the Linked Diet. You can email me at laurakopecwellness@gmail.com

ABOUT THE AUTHOR

Laura Kopec, NDT, MHNE, MA, CNC

Laura received a degree in Traditional Naturopathy from Trinity School of Natural Health, a Master of Science in Health and Nutrition Education from Hawthorn University, a Master of Arts from the University of Arizona, and a Nutritional Counseling Certificate from Trinity School of Natural Health.

Laura runs an educational consulting practice where she sees clients in person and by phone. She is available for speaking engagements and workshops/lectures. She is the author of *Let's Get Real About Eating: A practical guide to nutrition and health.* ISBN: 978-1-4525-7427-1 and *My Kids a Picky Eater: 12 Secrets to Changing Your Child's Eating Habits* ISBN: 978-1-5043-2656-8. For more information about Laura visit her website at www.laurakopec.com